Fight the Flab

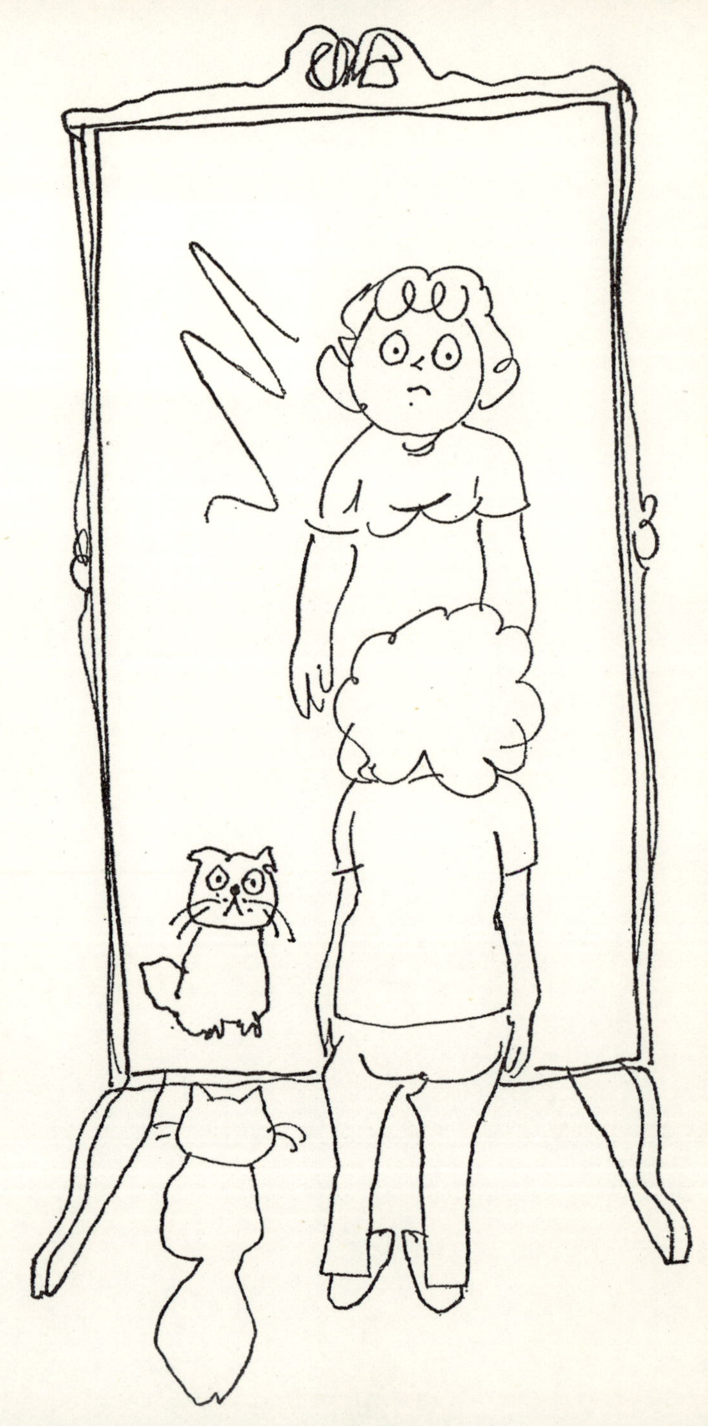

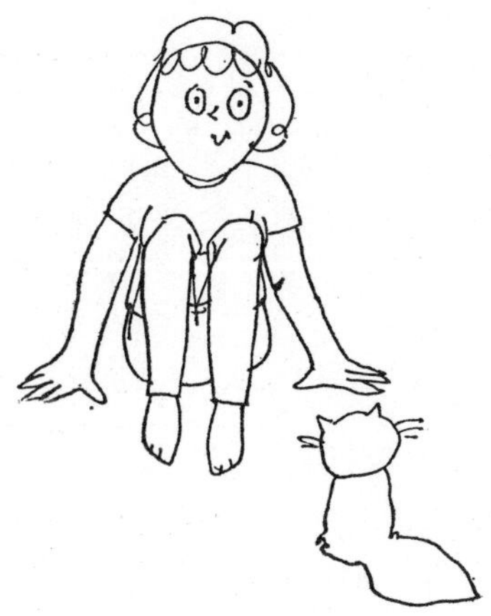

# Fight the Flab

## keep fit with

*Terry Wogan*

British Broadcasting Corporation

Published by the British Broadcasting Corporation,
35 Marylebone High Street, London WIM 4AA

SBN 563 11993 4

First published 1971



Printed in England by Cox and Wyman Ltd, London,
Reading and Fakenham

# Contents

# Introduction

When we started the 'Fight the Flab'
Battle of the Bulge or, as a French
listener has described it, 'Bataille de la
Brioche', in January 1970 in the Terry
Wogan Show on Radios 1 and 2, it was
with no high-flown motive of reducing
the Gross National Figure. The object
of the exercises was to hold our
listeners' attention, keep them amused –
revive their sagging interest if you like.

Very soon, however, it became apparent
that to many listeners 'Fight the Flab'
was no gimmick, but an important
activity to be pursued every day at
4 o'clock. Listeners write of how they
drop everything from hot irons to
husbands' dinners to join the good fight
and I get regular progress reports from
factory floors up and down the country
on the weekly weight loss.

The words 'Keep Fit' have always
seemed to me too imperative, too
tight-lipped and serious. My daily 'Fight
the Flab' is a light-hearted way of toning

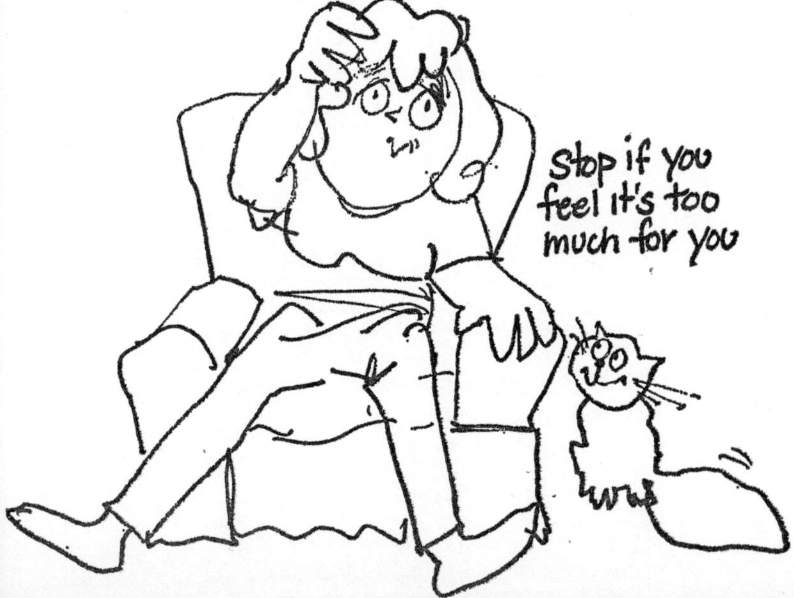

up, but none the less beneficial for that. Remember though, there is no need to corpse yourself. . . Stop if you feel any strain.

These exercises are all simple ones designed to help tone up your body and make you supple again.

Remember that you will be using a lot of muscles that are not accustomed to being exercised. So take it easy at first and gradually, as your body gets used to it, you can do more each day.

If you are in any doubt about exercising do not hesitate to consult your doctor.

These exercises alone will not make you lose weight but are excellent for toning up the muscles – especially when you are on a diet.

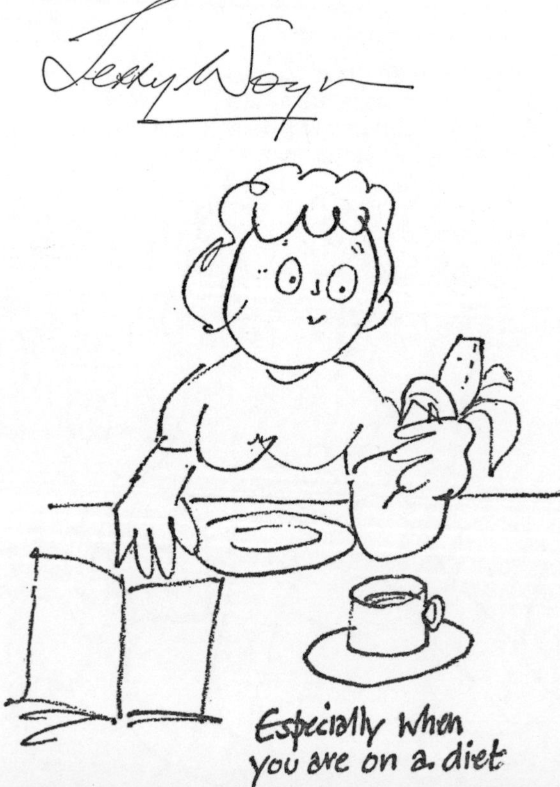

# 1 Limbering up 1

Before you do your specific exercises, try these limbering-up exercises to get the circulation going and for general fitness.

Try hopping twice on each foot alternately, then change to running on the spot and then back to hopping again.

Keep on your toes all the time – don't make any noise with your feet.

Stop when you feel you are getting puffed.

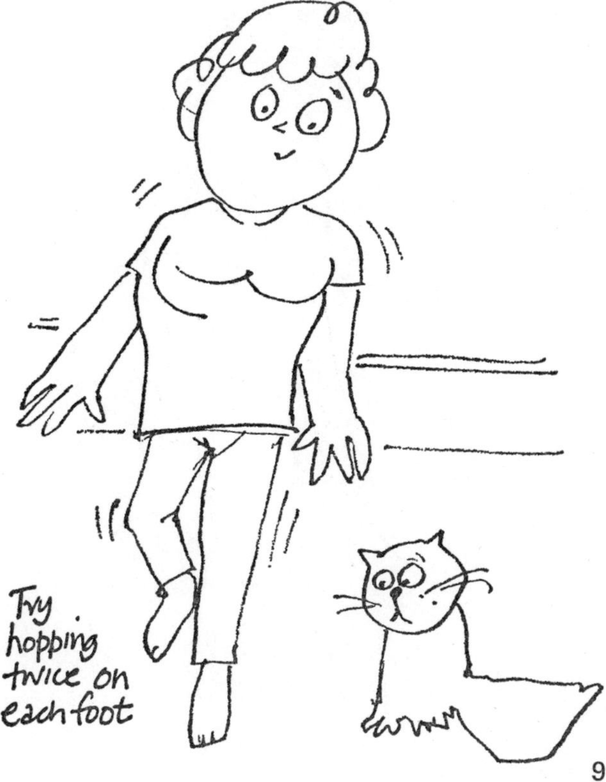

# 2 Limbering up 2

This time, try relaxing your arms and
shaking first the right arm – feel it go
limp – then the left.

Now shake the right leg and then the
left.

Now shake both arms and all of your
body.

Relax like a rag doll, bend from the
waist and trail your hands and wrists on
the floor.

Bend your knees, lift your arms up
above your head and stretch. Stand on
tiptoe and make yourself as tall as
possible.

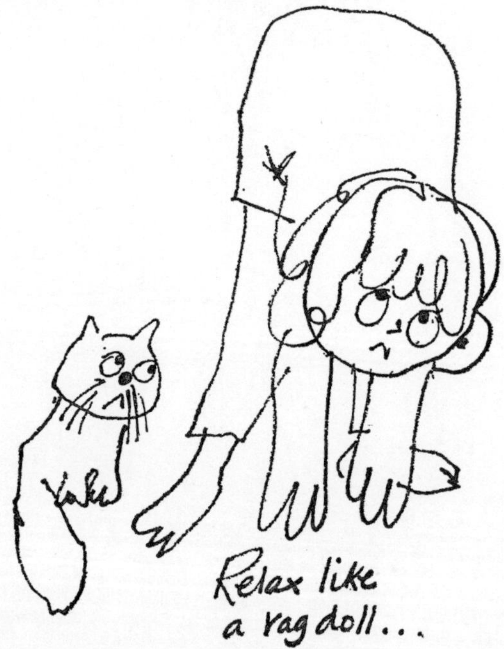

# 3 Learning how to breathe properly

When you have finished limbering up or exercising it is important to learn how to control your breathing.

You may find, too, that if you have been doing one or two rather strenuous exercises, you will be in need of a breather. Here's how to relax.

If you've been doing a standing-up exercise and you want to relax, bend your knees slightly, tuck your tail and tummy in, breathe in, stand up straight and breathe out.

If you've been lying down doing an exercise, relax by bending your knees, keeping your feet flat on the floor, hands comfortably on your tummy. Take a deep breath in and then breathe out.

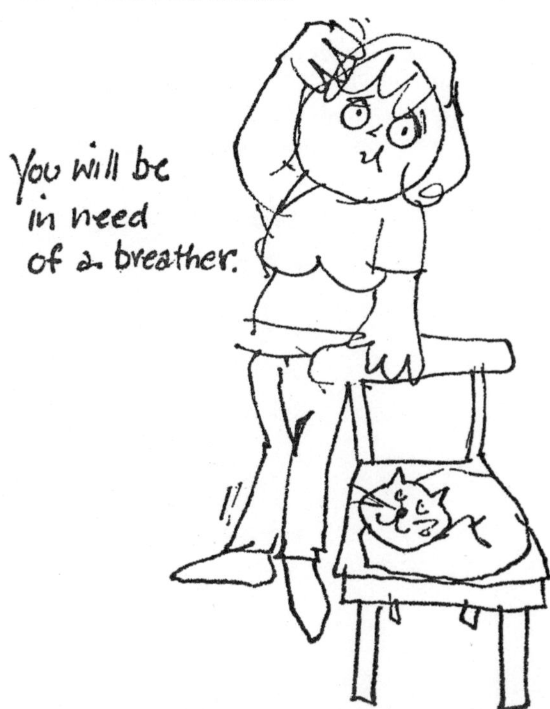

# 4 Good posture

This exercise teaches you how to stand well, and how to get down on to the floor correctly and up again.

For good posture it is important to learn how to stand and walk well. So: feet together, back straight, head up and arms loosely at your sides. Walk tall, hold your head up and look as if you own the ground that you are walking on!

To get down on to the floor to begin the exercises that you will be doing, first stand well, then kneel on one knee, then kneel on both knees, lower your body and place your right hand on the floor to your right side, sit on your right side and bring your legs round to the front. You are now ready to begin your exercises.

To get up again: bring your legs round to the side, kneel up on both knees, then up on one knee and stand up.

Adapt these movements to suit all the exercises and you will learn poise and grace.

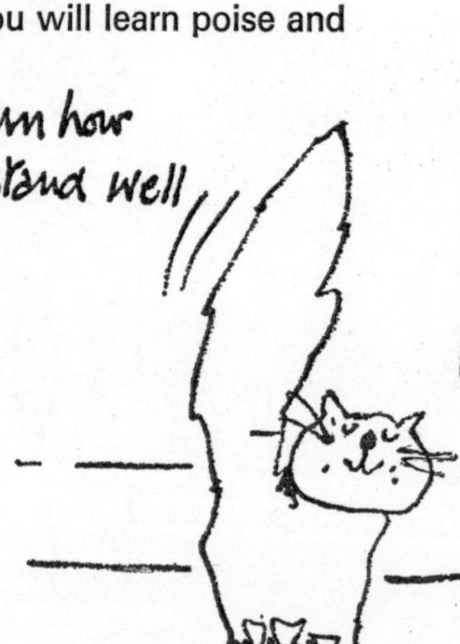

# 5 Neck muscles

Sit for this exercise.

Slowly and deliberately turn your
head to the right, now to the front, now
to the left.

Now – eyes front. Drop your head so
that your chin is resting on your chest;
then raise your head so that your eyes
are looking straight ahead and now
drop your head back.

Repeat these sequences three times
each.

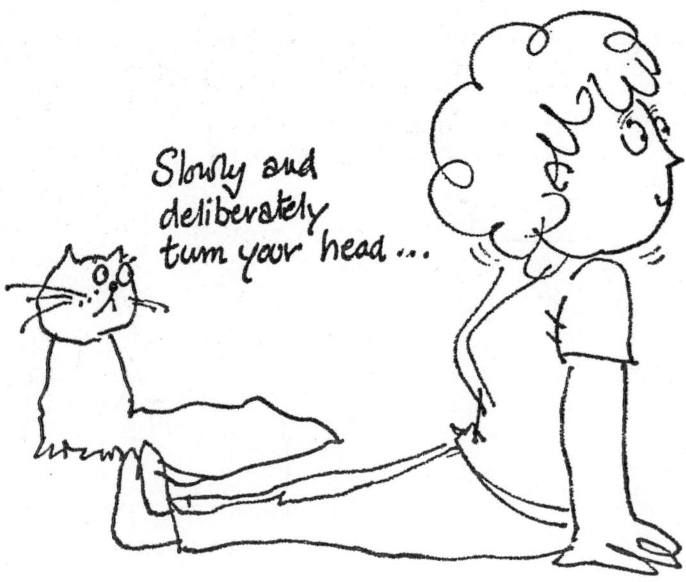

# 6 Facial muscles

This is a very easy exercise as you are
sitting down and all you need is a
mirror to make sure that you are doing
this properly.

As you are sitting, watch your posture;
keep your back straight – no slumping!

Now say a long exaggerated eeee and then
a long exaggerated oooo at the mirror
and watch yourself making these faces.

Try this exercise about ten times.

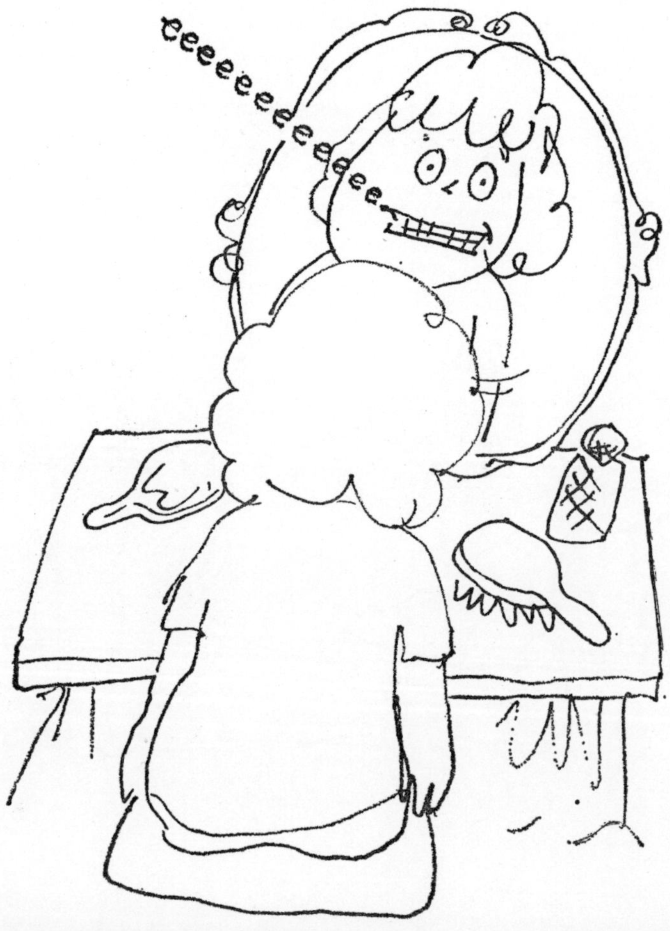

# **7** Fingers, hands and wrists

You can either sit or stand for the
following exercise, which is particularly
good for people like typists.

Start with your hands in front of you
in the air. Now clench both hands
tightly. Unclench them quickly
spreading your fingers wide with a
slight flicking action.

Start by doing this exercise about five
times but take it easy, or you will make
your hands ache.

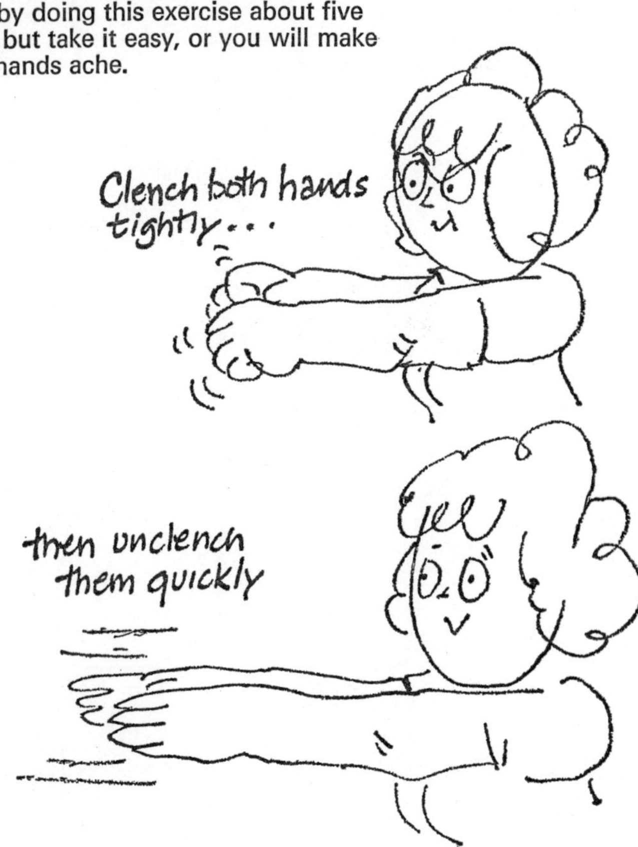

## 8 Hands and wrists

With your hands in front of you in the
air, let them hang loose at the wrist.
Now make a circling movement with
your fingertips.

Try to combine exercise 7 – clenching
and unclenching your hands and
spreading your fingertips wide – with
the above exercise.

Do exercise 7 about five times, then
carry straight on to exercise 8, doing
this also about five times.

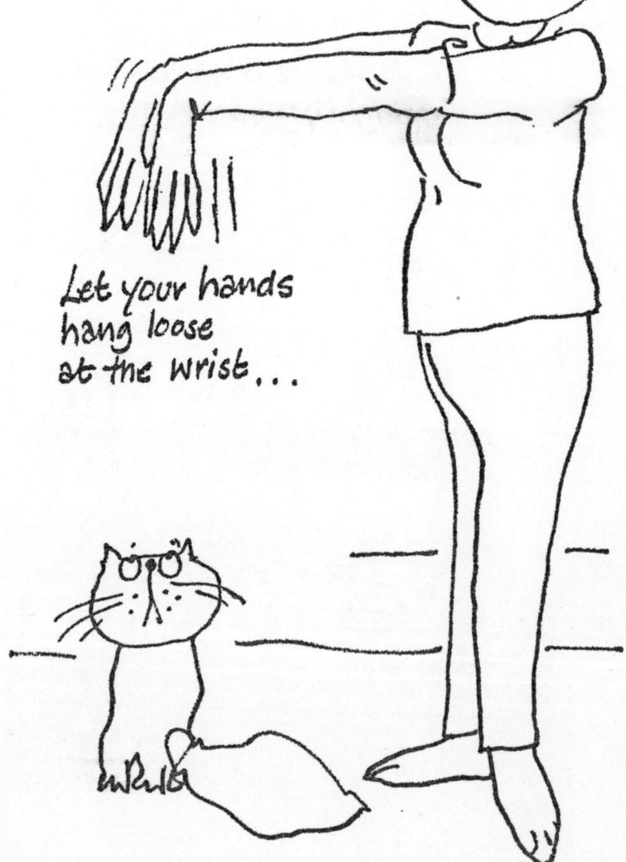

# 9 How to gain slim, trim ankles

You can sit for this exercise and it is best to take your shoes off so that you aren't restricted.

Take hold of your right ankle with both hands and place your right leg across your left one.

Point your toes and make a circling movement with your foot.

Try this circling movement half a dozen times, then repeat it with your left ankle.

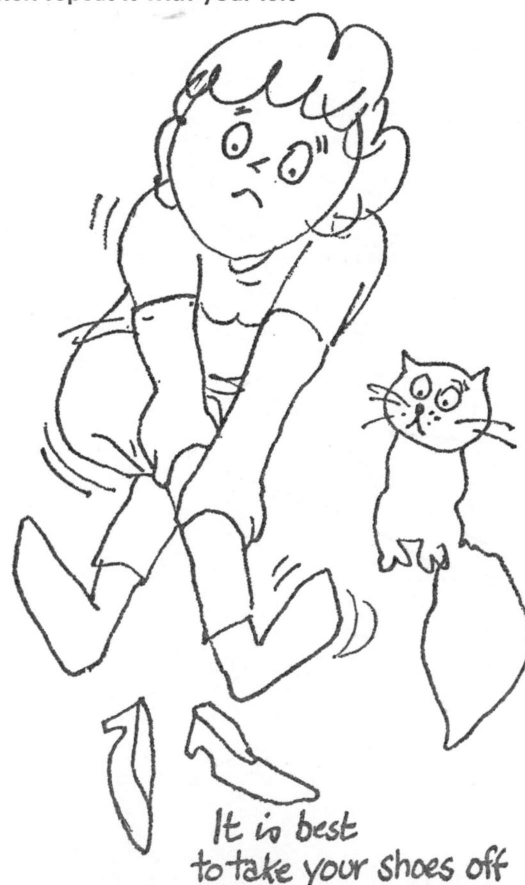

## **10** Feet, ankles and posture

Sit on the floor with your legs straight
out in front of you, flat on the floor,
heels about one foot apart.

Move your feet so that your toes make
large circling movements. Press out,
and around and in towards your body.
Don't take your feet off the floor.

Try this exercise moving your toes in
one direction for the count of five –
one complete circle counts as one –
then change direction again for the
count of five.

Stop if you feel any strain.

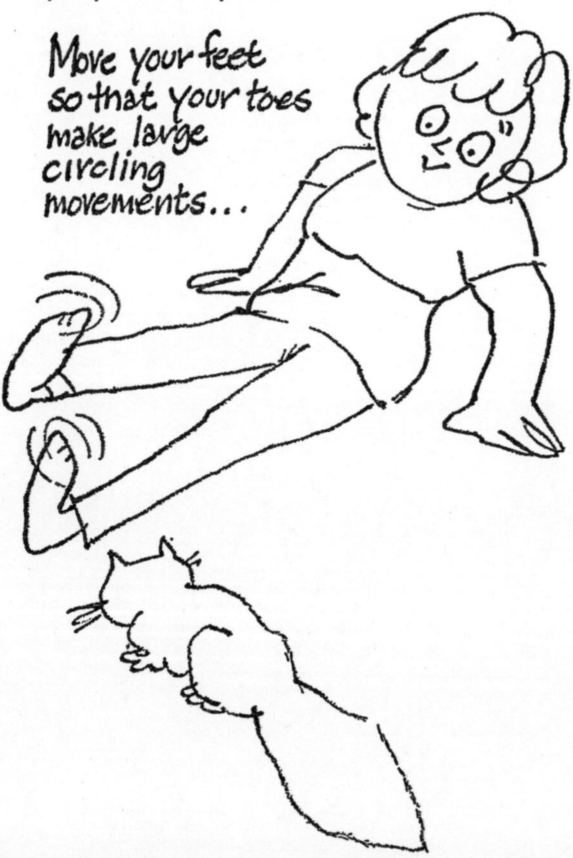

# 11 Feet, ankles and calves

Stand well: head up, back straight, arms loosely at your sides and feet slightly apart.

Very slowly, raise yourself up on to tiptoe and hold for a count of three. Then slowly lower again until feet are flat on the floor.

Repeat four times to begin with and gradually increase, stopping if you feel any strain.

To help you keep your balance whilst on tiptoe, try pressing the sides of your heels together.

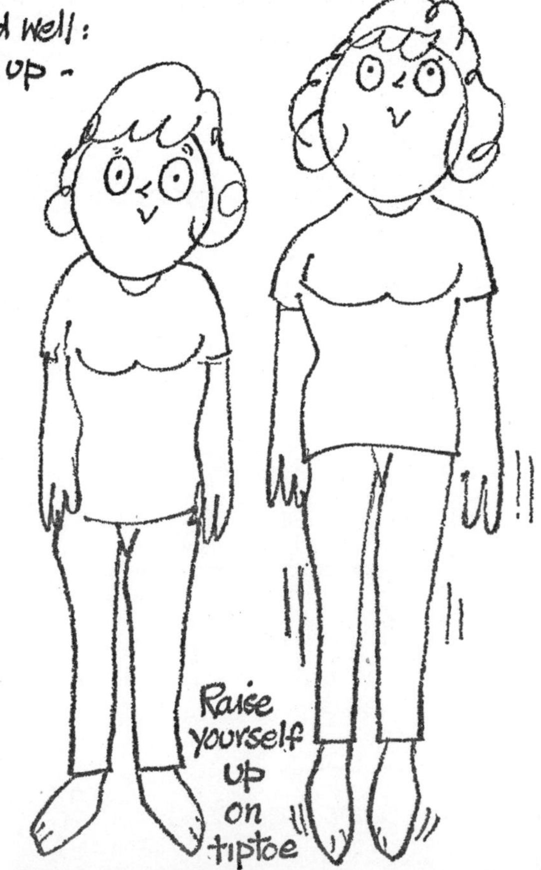

# 12 Toe wriggling

Sit on the floor with your legs straight out in front of you.

Begin with your heels on the floor. Now point your toes towards the ceiling, then point them towards the wall.

Repeat this movement – to the ceiling then to the wall–five times.

Now stop, wriggle your toes for the count of five, then continue pointing them.

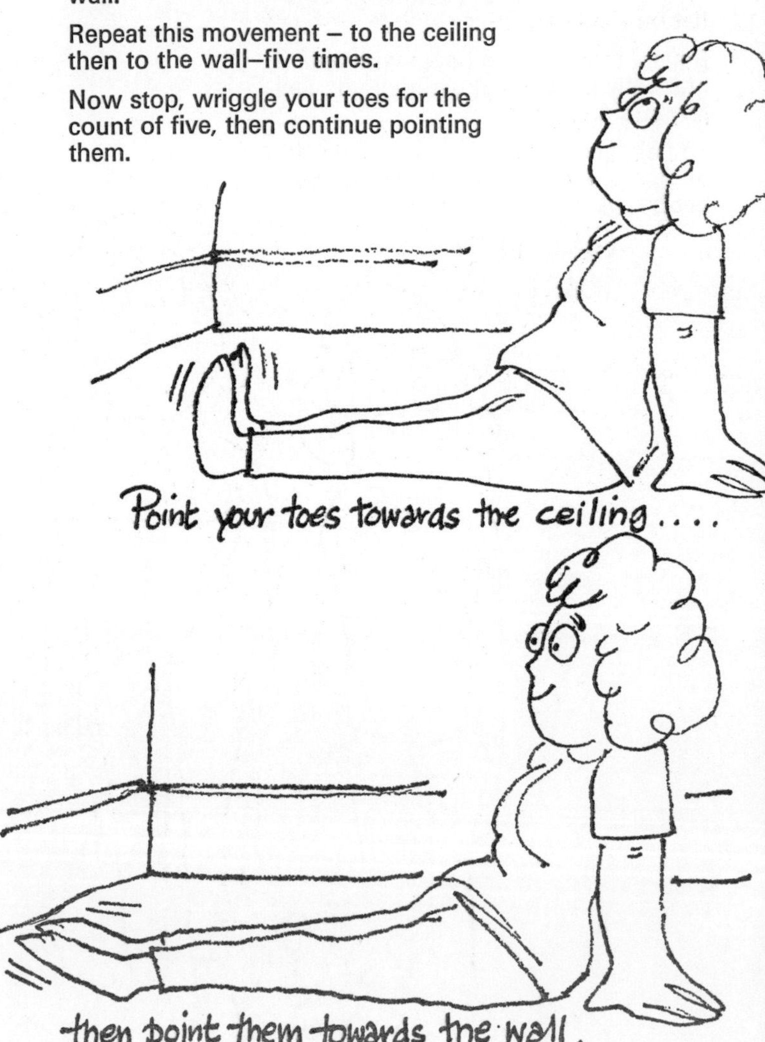

# 13 Chest muscles

Stand for this exercise with your feet
about one foot apart.

Keeping both arms straight, swing
them both in front of you and clap, then
swing them both behind you and clap.

Repeat eight times, but stop if you feel
any strain.

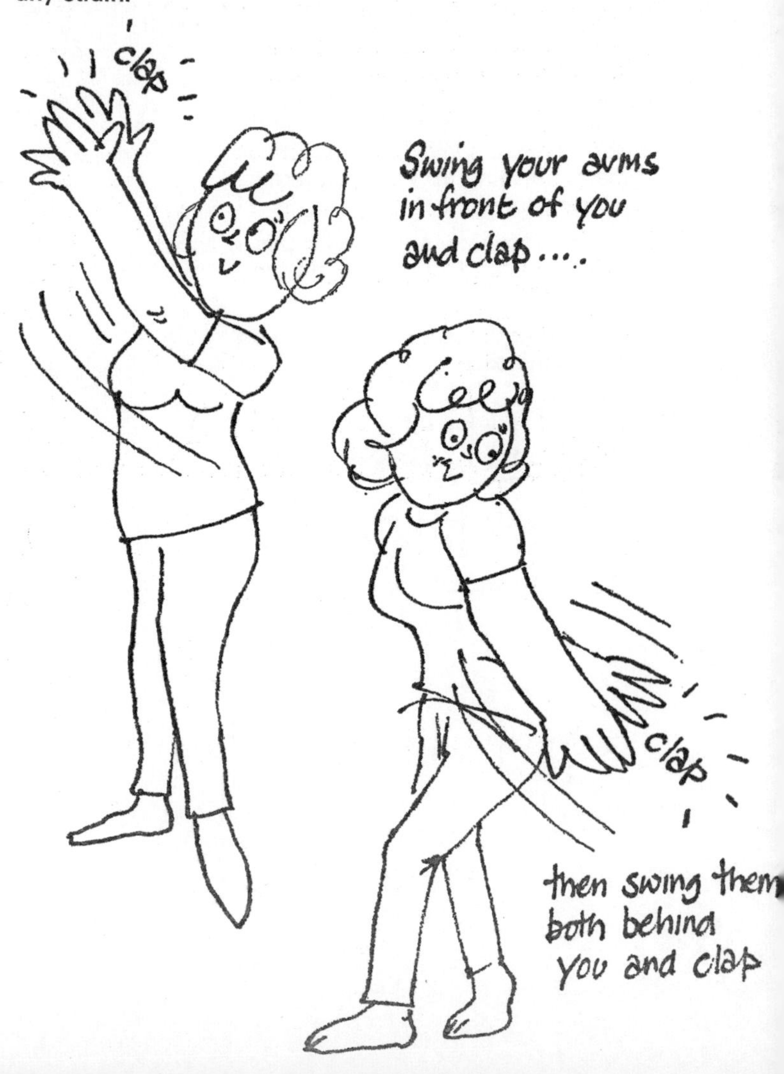

## **14** Upper arm and chest muscles

For this exercise you need to find two books of approximately the same size and weight.

Stand well and make sure you have a good area around you so that you can fling your arms about without any danger of banging into anything.

Take one book in each hand. Start with your arms down by your side. Raise both arms at once straight in front of you and swing them up and back and make a large circle with each of them, finishing up with your arms down by your side.

Stop if you feel any strain. With this exercise you can feel the pull on the muscles at the tops of your arms.

Start with six times for both arms and gradually increase.



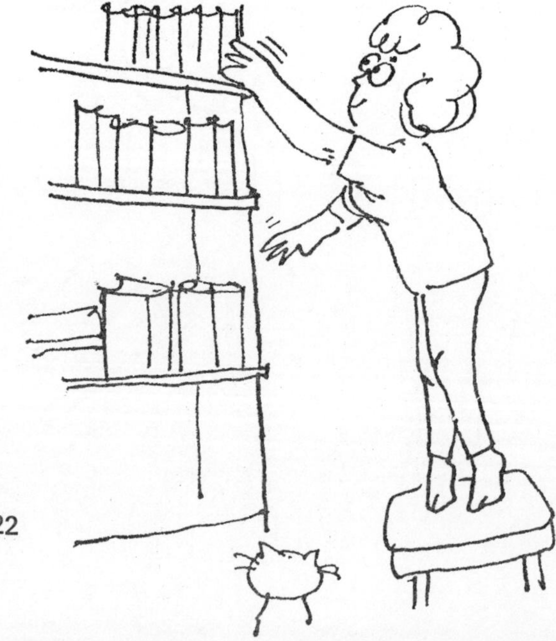

## **15** Neck, shoulders and bust

You can either sit or stand for this exercise.

Keeping your right arm straight down by your side, lift your right shoulder-blade up and make a circling movement. Repeat with left shoulder.

This is a very soothing way of easing aching or tense shoulder muscles.

Remember your posture when you are doing this exercise. Either sit or stand up straight.

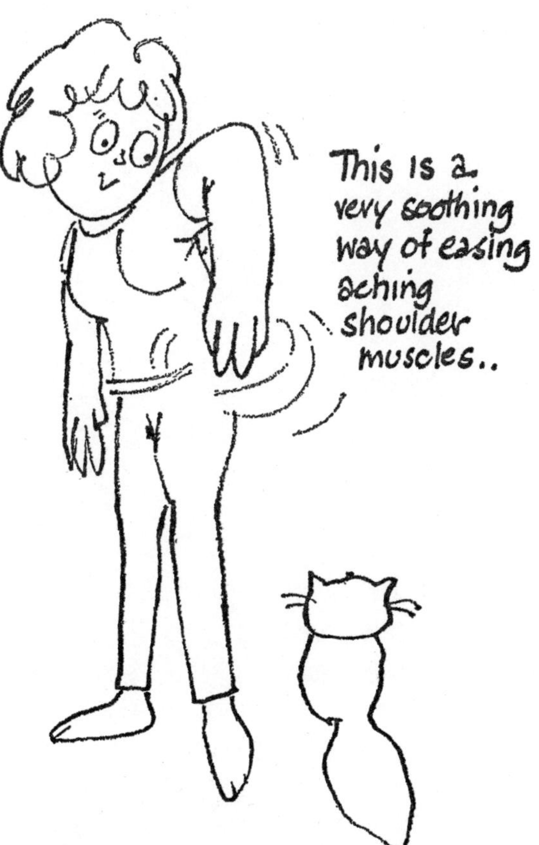

# 16 The waist 1

First stand well, then get down on to
the floor as in exercise 4. Your legs
should be straight out in front of you
ready for the exercise.

Bending forward from the waist, using
both hands, touch the floor lightly with
your fingertips by your right foot then
by your left foot. Then touch the floor
with your fingertips lightly by your right
knee and then by your left. Lastly,
swing your hands as far round to your
right side as you can and touch the
floor and then to your left. Get a really
good swing on this last movement.

Finish your exercise properly, stand
up – and stand well.

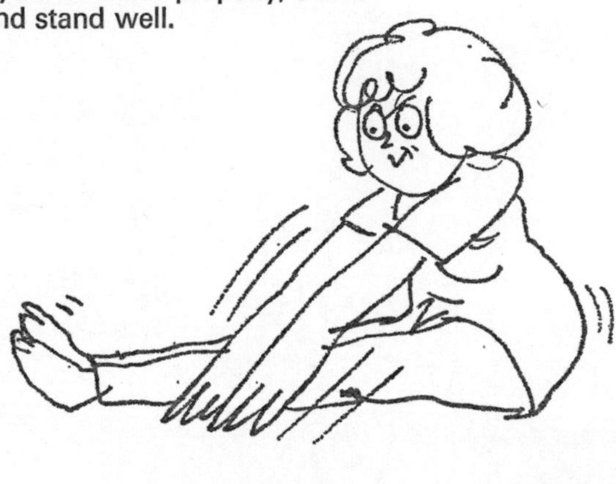

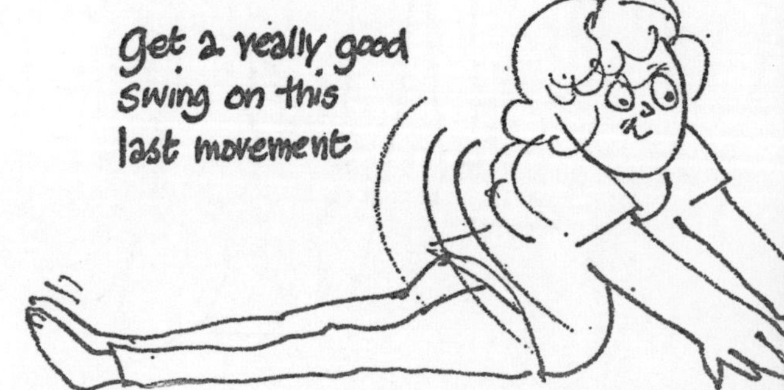

# 17 The waist 2

Stand well, feet comfortably apart.

Clasp your hands together in front of
you. Twist them round as far as you
can to the right, with one hand, as it
were, pulling the other one round.
Repeat to the left.

Then try this exercise with your hands
clasped at head level, twisting from
right to left.

The object of this exercise is to get a
good swing with your body and feel
the pull on your waist.

Finish your exercise by standing well.

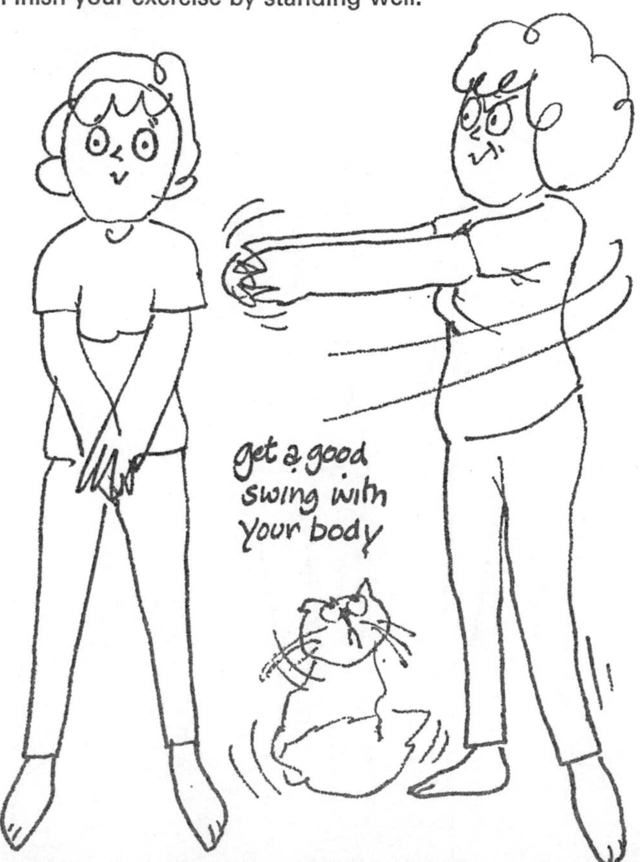

## **18** The waist 3

Stand well, feet comfortably apart.

Raise your right arm, until it is straight
above your head and close to your ear.

With your left arm, creep your hand
slowly down your left leg as far as you
can.

Bend your body and feel the pull on
your right side.

Repeat with the opposite side.

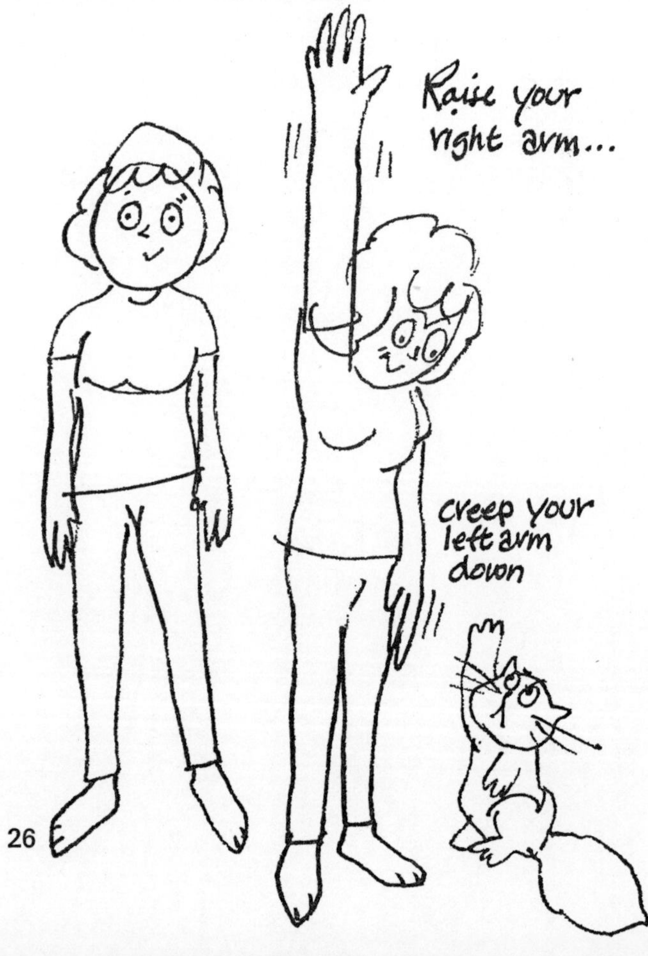

# 19 The waist and upper arms

Stand with your feet comfortably apart.
Raise your arms straight up in the air
and clasp your hands together.

Moving to the right, make a large circle
in front of you with your hands still
clasped, till you come back to where
you started with your arms straight
above your head.

Moving to the left, make a large circle
till your arms are straight up above your
head again.

Repeat to the right again – and so on.

Feel the pull on your waist and make
sure you keep your arms as extended
as possible.

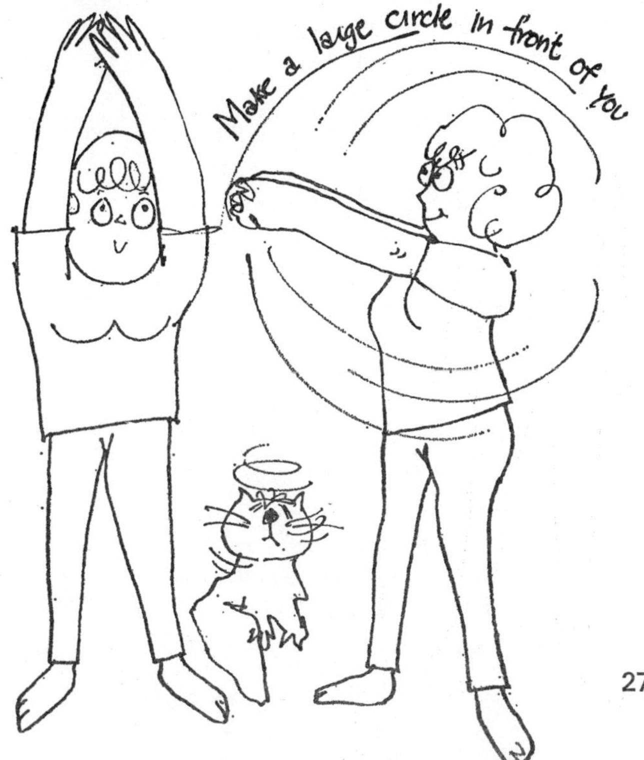


27

## **20** The waist and hips

For this exercise you will need to be
kneeling on the floor in an upright
position, not sitting back on your heels.
Fold your arms in front of you.

Still keeping your arms folded and your
back as straight as you can, sit on the
floor, first to your right side, then return
to your upright kneeling position and
then sit to your left side.

This exercise is rather hard on the
knees, but as you are doing it you can
feel the pull on your waist and your
back stretching.

Start this exercise three times each
side, finishing in the upright kneeling
position so that you can get up
comfortably. Stop, however, should
you feel any strain.

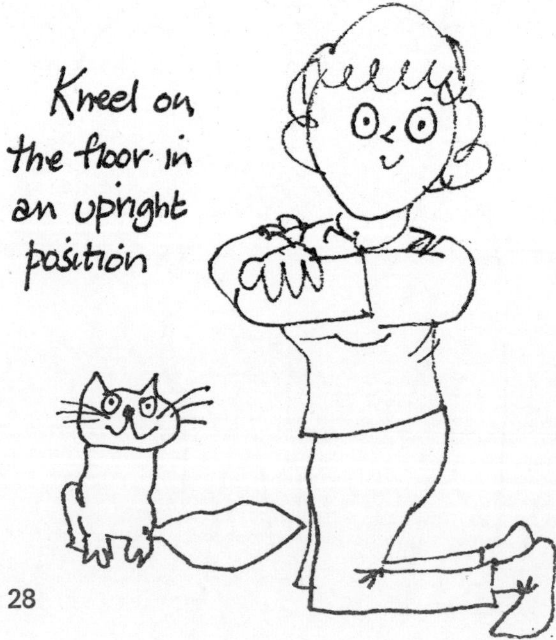

# 21 Waist, hips and back

Get down on to the floor, so that you are on your hands and knees. Make sure that the palms of your hands are flat on the floor in a direct line under your shoulders and your knees are directly under your hips.

Hump your back, letting your head fall between your arms. Now straighten up, straighten your back, with your head up, looking at the wall in front of you.

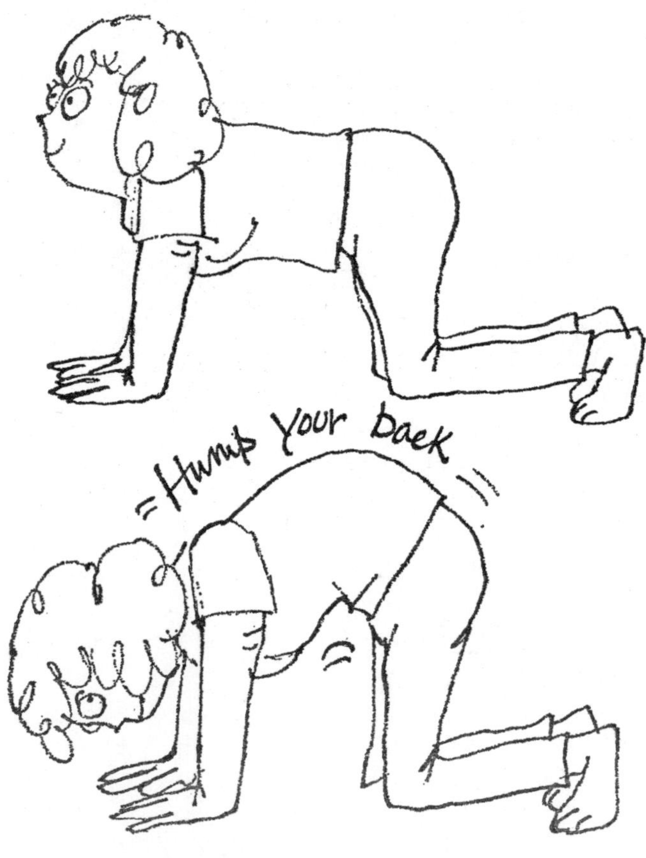

## **22** Back, waist and hips

For this exercise you will need a
dining-room or kitchen chair with a
reasonably straight back and no arms.

Start by sitting on the chair, with
your feet flat on the floor slightly apart.

Bend down and touch your toes and
let your head drop on to your knees.
Raise your head and body, lift your arms
straight up in the air and point your
fingertips. Tilt your head and look at
your fingertips. Get a good stretch on
this movement and feel the pull on your
waist. Bring your arms down and relax.

Repeat the whole movement five
times to begin with, if you can manage
this. Stop if you feel any strain.

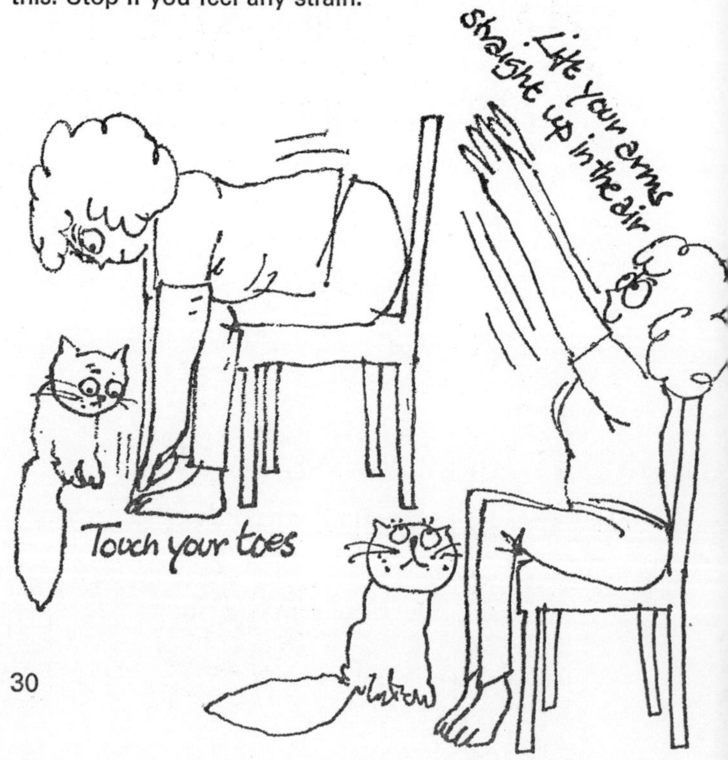

## 23 Waist, hips and legs

This is another sitting exercise using a
chair with no arms and a straight back.

Sit on the chair and hold the sides of
the chair seat with both hands. Keep
your feet together flat on the floor.

Bending your knee, lift your right leg
up, and point your toes. Put your right
leg down. Now bending your left knee,
lift it up and point your toes.

Keep your head up and shoulders back.

Start this exercise using three lifts of
each leg, and stop immediately if you
feel any strain.

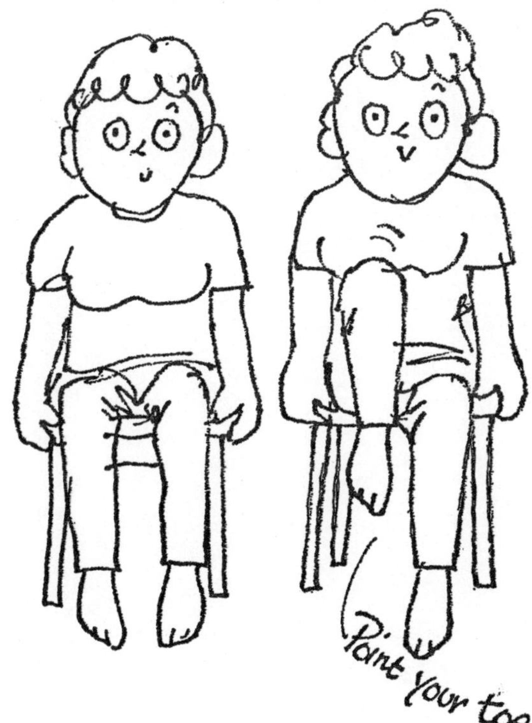

## 24 Waist and hips 1

Kneel down, with your hands on the
floor in front of you. Make sure that
the palms of your hands are flat on the
floor in a direct line under your shoulders
and your knees are directly under your
hips.

Swivel your hips to the right, at the
same time turning your head to look
back at your right hip. Now swivel your
hips to the left, turning your head to
look back at your left hip.

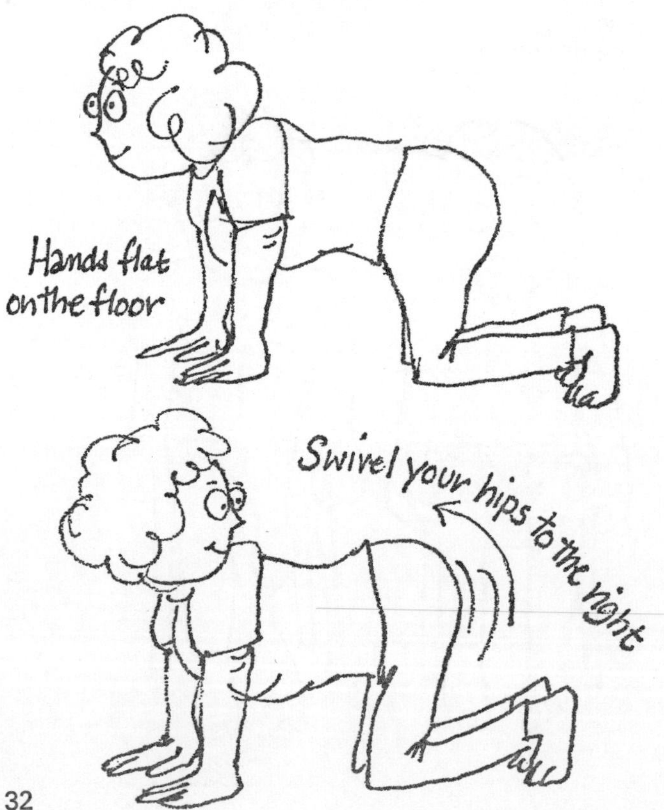

# 25 Waist and hips 2

Kneel down, with your hands on the floor in front of you. Make sure that the palms of your hands are flat on the floor in a direct line under your shoulders and your knees are directly under your hips.

Begin by slowly bending your right knee towards your chest, putting your foot flat on the floor. Drop your head and let your forehead rest on your knee. Make sure that you keep your hands flat on the floor at all times.

With a swift movement, stretch your right leg straight out behind you. Arch your back.

Relax, then repeat with the left leg.

Watch your poise and balance in this exercise. Keep your head up and your bottom tucked in while you are doing the stretching movement.

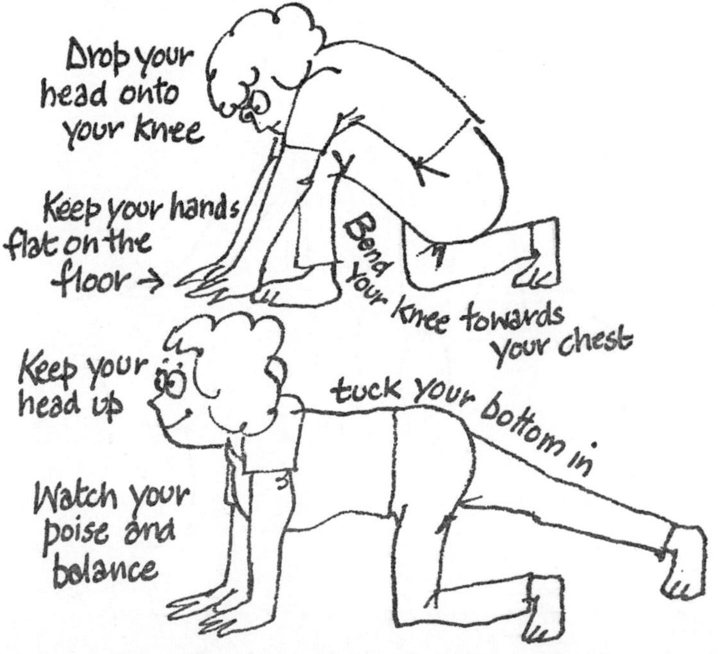

# 26 Hips and waist

For this exercise you will need to be
sitting on the floor with both your knees
comfortably bent towards your chest,
and your arms out to the side of you
with the palms of your hands face
downwards on the floor.

Keep your back straight. Now in three
positive movements, lower your knees
to the right-hand side of you until they
are resting on the floor. Return them so
that they are in front of you, now lower
them both to your left-hand side and
then raise them until you are back in
your starting position again.

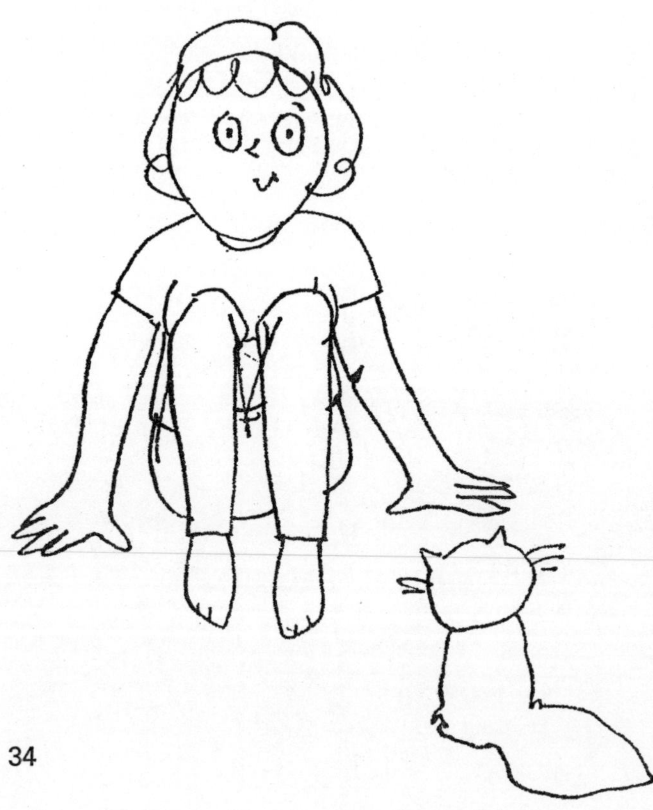

# **27** Waist and thighs

For this exercise you will need a chair
with a straight back and no arms.

Sit on the chair and begin with your
feet together and flat on the floor.
Hold the back of the chair.

Raise both knees up together off the
floor and point your toes. Put your legs
down slowly. Repeat five times.

Watch your posture on this exercise
and sit with your back straight and head
up. No slumping or round shoulders!

Stop if you feel the slightest strain.

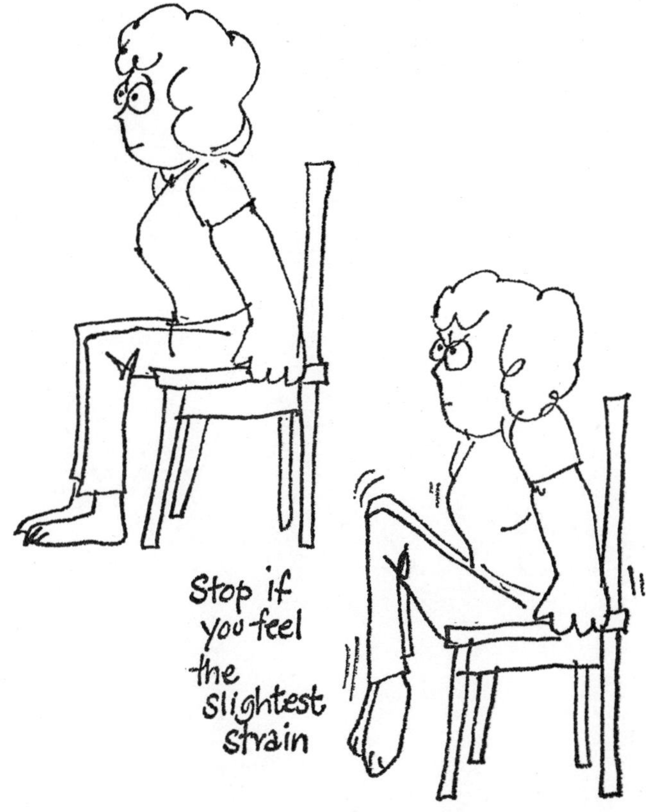

# 28 Back muscles

Lie on your back on the floor, knees comfortably bent, feet flat on the floor, with your arms by your side, palms face downward.

Pressing down on the floor with the palms of your hands, arch your back.

Relax and let your spine press down on the floor. If you are doing this exercise properly, you will have a flat stomach too!

Repeat three times to begin with and gradually increase.

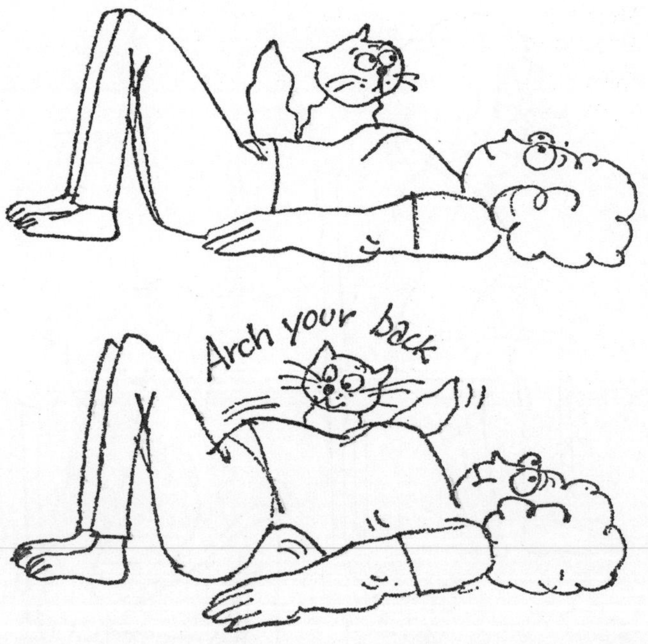

# 29 Back and hips

Sit on the floor with your legs straight
out in front of you. Your arms should be
straight and to the back of you, with the
palms of your hands face downwards,
flat on the floor.

Keeping your heels on the floor, raise
your hips up from the floor, using your
arms to support you. Now cross your
right leg over your left one, swinging it
as far over as possible. Return your
right leg. Now cross your left leg over
your right leg, swinging it as far over
as possible. Lower your hips on the
floor again and sit down.

Repeat this complete movement three
times to begin with.

This exercise is quite strenuous so stop
if you feel any strain.

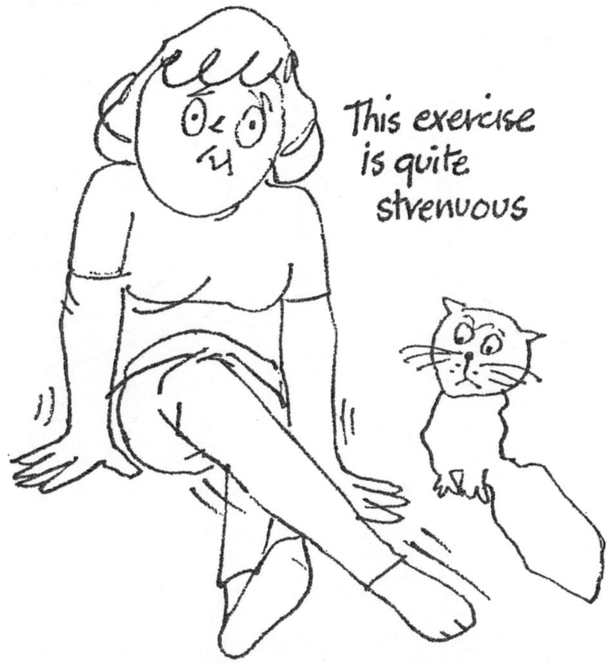

## **30** Back, waist and legs

Lie flat on your stomach with your
elbows and hands on the floor, palms
face downwards. Tuck your toes under.
Don't fully extend your arms but use
your elbows as a prop.

Lift your hips and shoulders up from the
floor and hold for a count of three.
Make sure that you have a straight line
from head to toe.

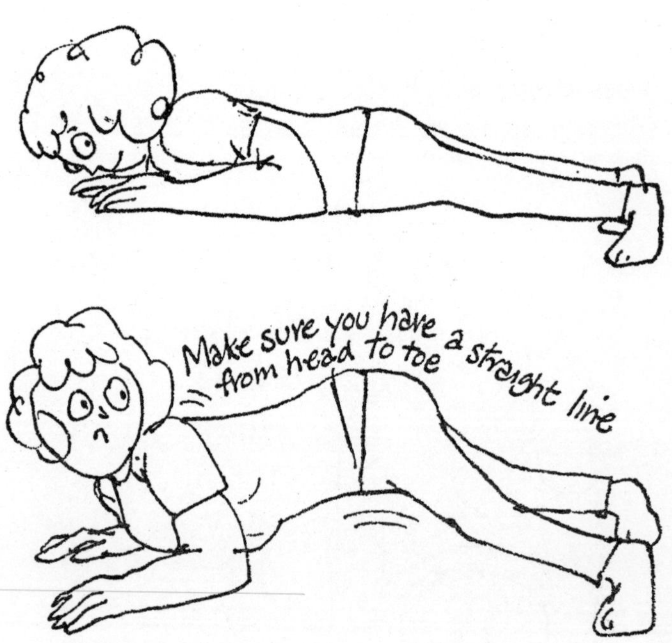

# 31 General fitness

Get down on to the floor. Lie flat on
your back with the palms of your hands
face downwards at your side, knees
bent, feet flat on the floor.

With a swift movement, press on the
palms of your hands, raise your legs
together and swing them up and over
your head, so that you finish up with
the tips of your toes resting on the
floor behind your head. Then roll back.

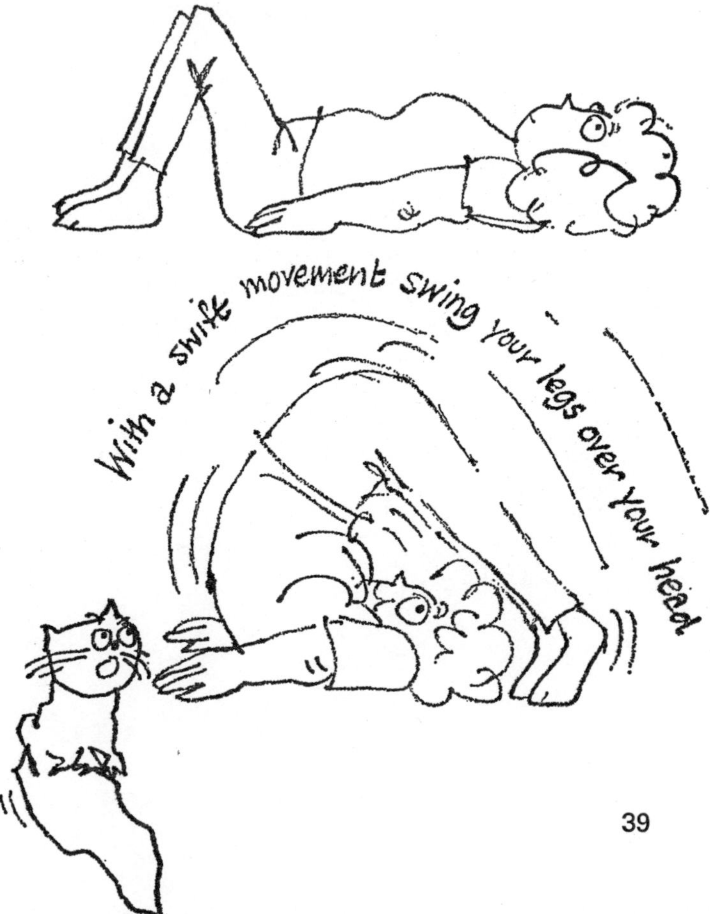

## 32 Stomach, back and general fitness

Begin your exercise by standing well.
Get down on to the floor and roll over
on to your stomach.

Grasp both of your ankles with your
hands and try to pull your head and
chest up from the floor.

Try this exercise at first three times.
In between each heave, relax and rest
your chin on the floor.

Finish your exercise by getting up from
the floor, remembering your posture.

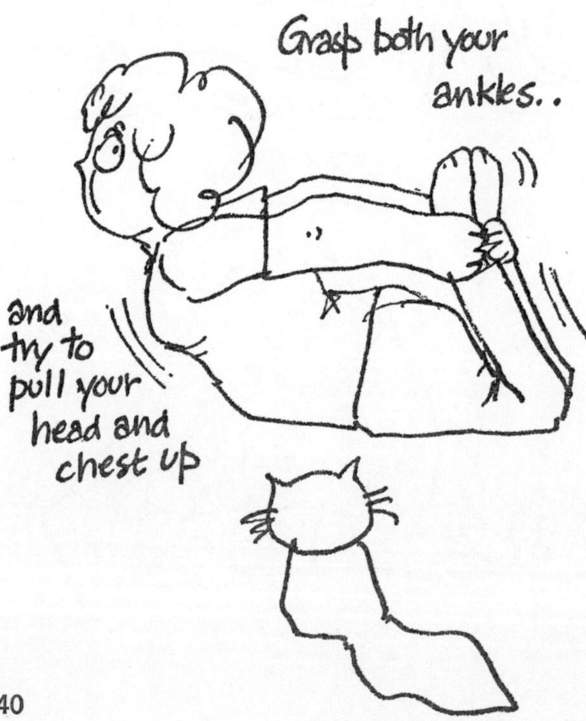

# **33** Stomach and thigh muscles 1

Lie flat on your back on the floor, arms out to the side, palms face downwards.

Without bending your right leg, raise it straight up in the air. Now stretch it over to your left side and try and touch your left hand with your right foot.

Still keeping your leg straight, lift it up in the air again, then lower it back to the ground.

Now try this with your left leg over to your right side and try and touch your right hand with your left foot.

*No cheating* – keep your shoulders flat on the floor!

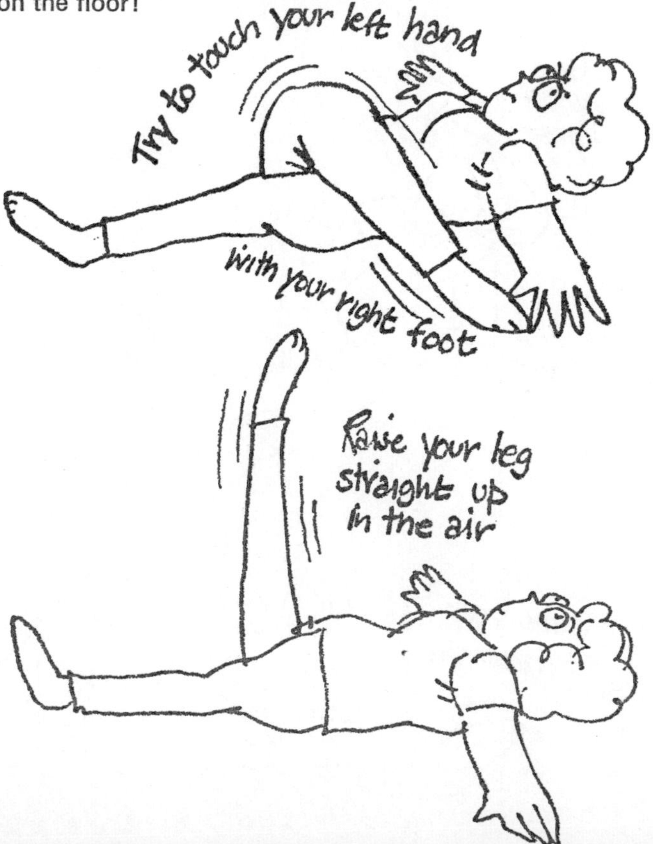

# **34** Stomach and thigh muscles 2

Get down on to the floor. Sit with your legs together out on the floor in front of you, hands on the floor, palms face downwards, comfortably by your side.

Keeping your feet flat on the floor, slide both knees up together until they are under your chin. At the same time hug your knees with your arms.

Now let go of your knees, open your arms wide, arch your back and slide your feet down the floor, until your legs are straight again.

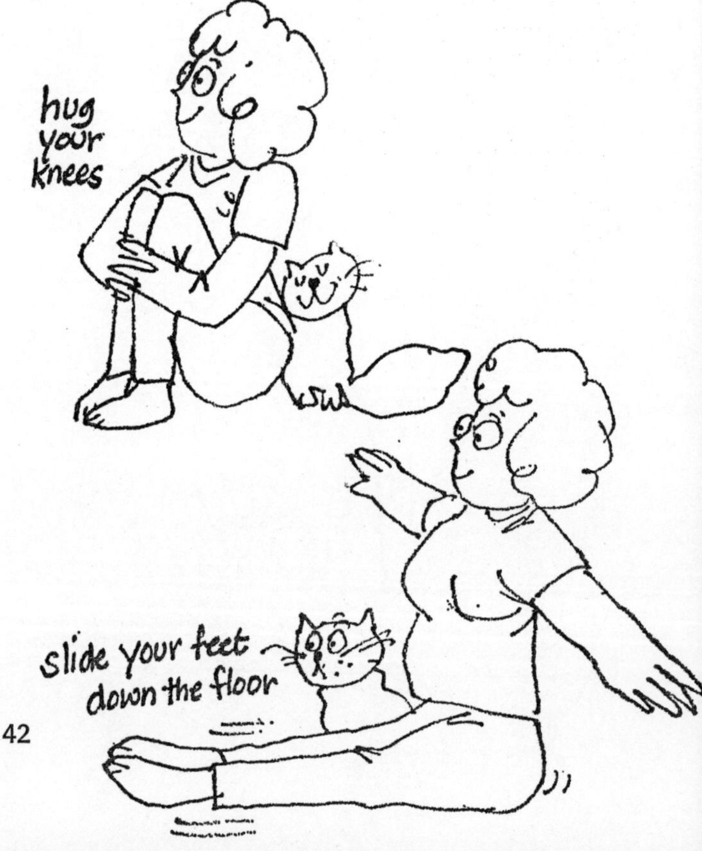

## 35 Stomach and thigh muscles 3

Get down on to the floor, lie on your left side, supporting your head with your left hand and elbow, legs straight out in front of you.

Keeping both legs together, bend your knees towards your chest, raising them off the ground slightly, then straighten your legs and relax. Repeat this three times on your left side and then turn over and repeat three times on your right side.

With this exercise, feel the pull on your stomach. You may find it helps you to balance better if you put your other hand flat on the floor just in front of you.

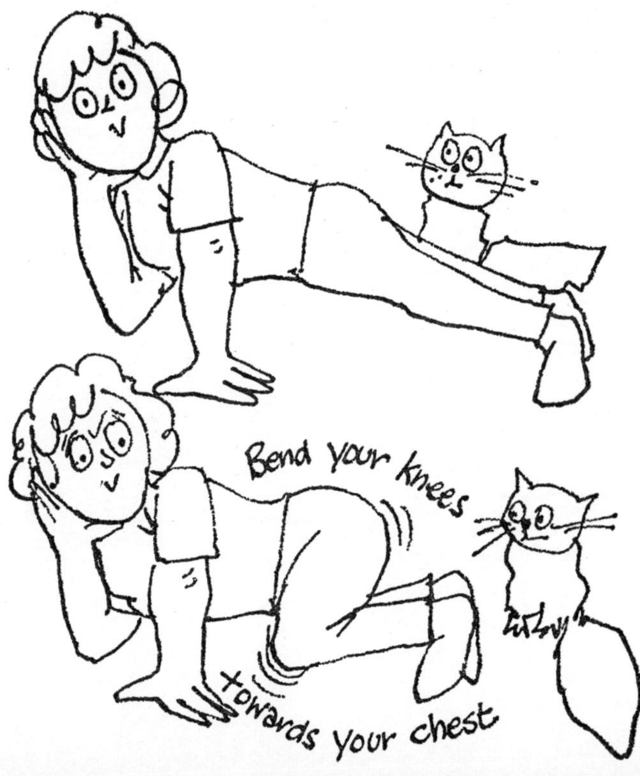

# 36 Stomach, back and thighs

For this exercise you need to be lying
flat out on your stomach. Fold your
arms and rest your head comfortably
on them.

Start by lifting your right leg slowly
straight up in the air behind you. Put it
down slowly. Now lift your left leg
slowly, remembering to keep it straight.
Lower your left leg slowly.

Repeat three times with each leg to
begin with, then see if you can gradually
increase. You must be very careful if
you are not used to exercising and stop
if you feel any strain whatsoever.
With this exercise you can feel the
muscles in the backs of your thighs
working.

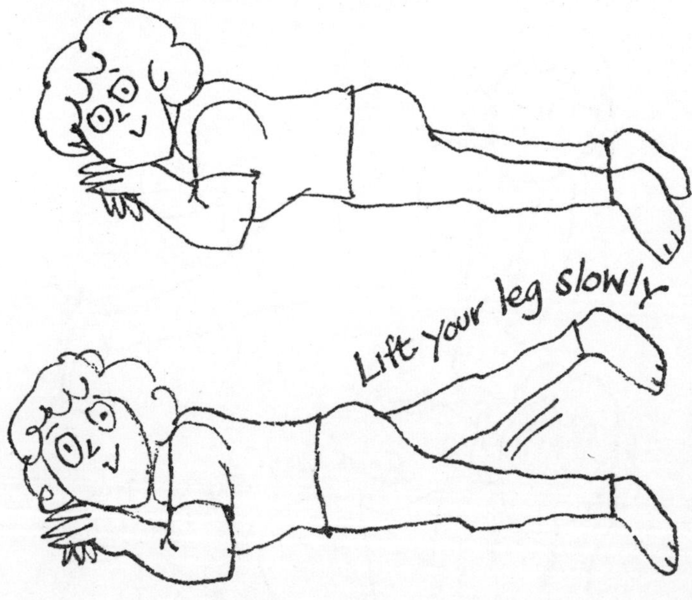

## 37 The stomach

Stand well and then get down on to the floor as you have been taught.

Lie flat on your back on the floor with hands comfortably at your sides, palms face downwards.

Bend both your knees up to your chest and then raise both legs up straight together.

Lower both legs as slowly as you can until they touch the floor, remembering to keep them straight.

You must be very careful not to strain your stomach muscles and stop if you feel it is too much for you. Try this exercise about twice first of all, then gradually increase when you feel your muscles are getting used to it.

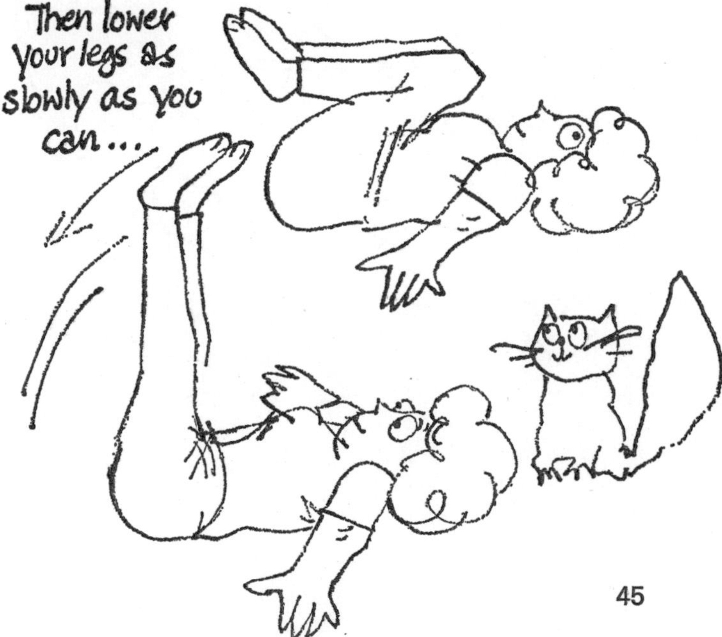

# 38 Stomach muscles 1

Stand well, then lie flat on your back
on the floor with your hands resting
on the front of your thighs.
Creep your hands down to your knees
at the same time lifting your head and
shoulders off the floor. Hold for the
count of three, and relax.
Repeat.

Don't forget to finish your exercise by
getting up and standing well for good
posture.

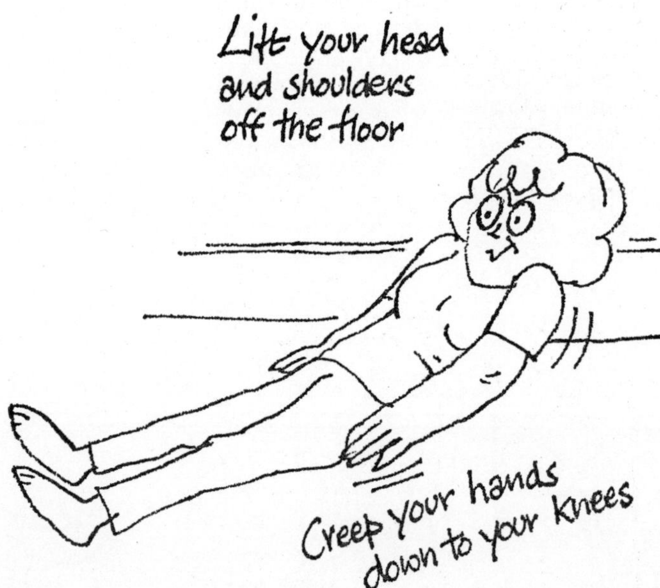

# 39 Stomach muscles 2

Lie flat on the floor, legs out straight, with your hands clasped together behind your head.

Now lift your head and shoulders up from the floor and try to reach a sitting position. Do not use your hands in any way – keep them behind your head and keep your legs out straight still on the floor.

If you find this exercise particularly difficult, try anchoring your feet under a wardrobe or a cupboard just to give yourself a bit of support, but don't bring the lot down on yourself. If you rise quickly from the floor you won't lose your balance.

Start by doing this exercise about three times. Be careful not to overdo it and stop if you feel any strain. Muscles not normally used have to be treated with care.

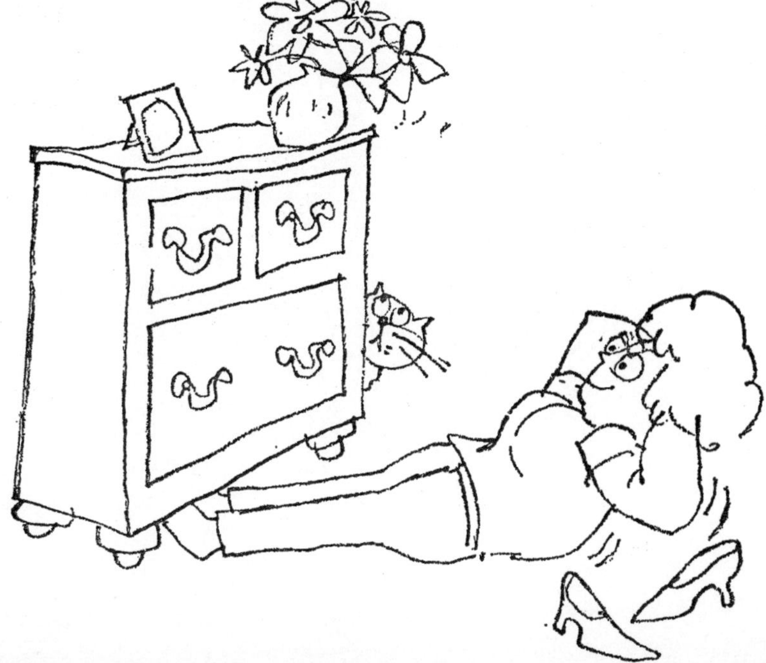

## **40** Stomach muscles 3

Get down on to the floor then lie flat on your back with your arms out to the side, palms face downwards.

Bend both knees to your chest and roll to the right, then stretch your legs out straight. Now bend your knees back to your chest and roll over to the left and stretch your legs fully again.

Start by doing this exercise twice on each side as it is quite strenuous and gradually increase it.

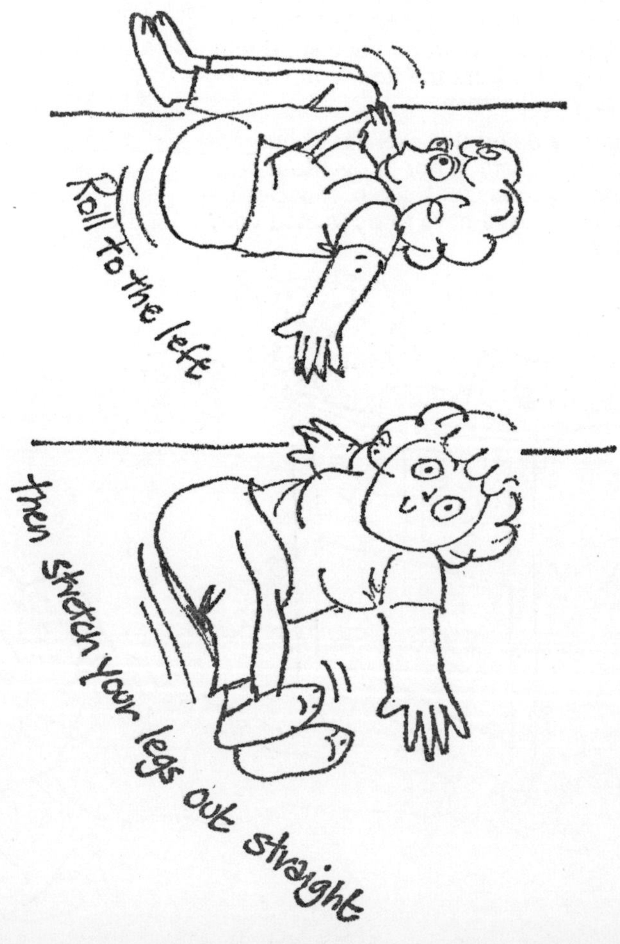

## **41** Bottom, stomach muscles and back

Sit on floor with your back straight. Put your legs out in front with your knees straight.

Keeping your arms loosely at each side, rock to the right, letting your right hand take your body-weight, then rock to the left, letting your left hand take your body-weight.

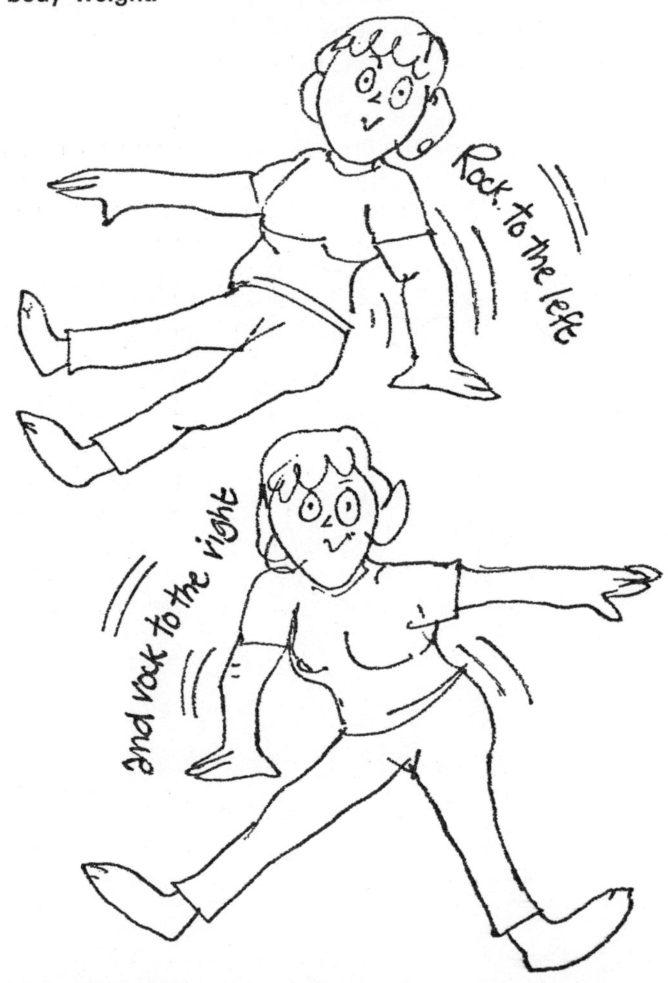

# **42** Stomach and back muscles

Begin the exercise by standing well,
feet comfortably apart.

Keeping your legs straight, bend from
the waist and try to touch the floor in
front of you with your fingertips.
Repeat five times.

When you have mastered this, try to
get the palms of your hands flat on the
floor in front of you. Bend and pat the
floor three times. Repeat this five times.

Finish your exercise by standing well.
Then bend your knees slightly, tuck
your tail and stomach in, and breathe
in, stand up straight and breathe out.

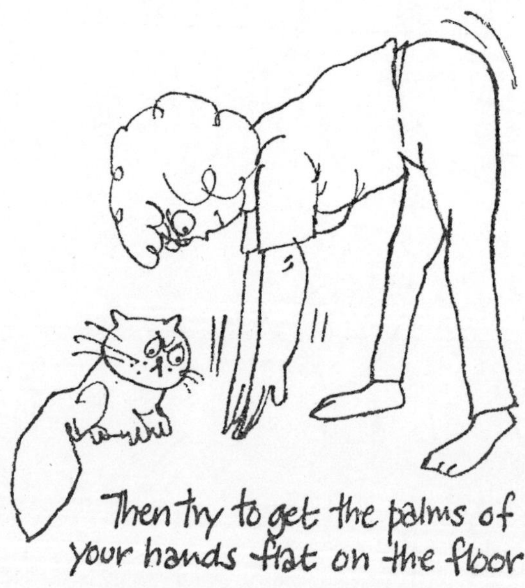

# **43** Stomach and thighs 1

For this exercise you will need to be
flat on your back on the floor, legs out
straight, with your arms out sideways
and the palms of your hands face
downwards on the floor.

Bend your right knee towards your
chest. Now raise your right leg straight
up in the air and point your toes, bend
your knee towards your chest again and
put your leg down.

Repeat with your left leg.

Do this exercise six times each leg to
begin with, but do stop if you feel any
strain.

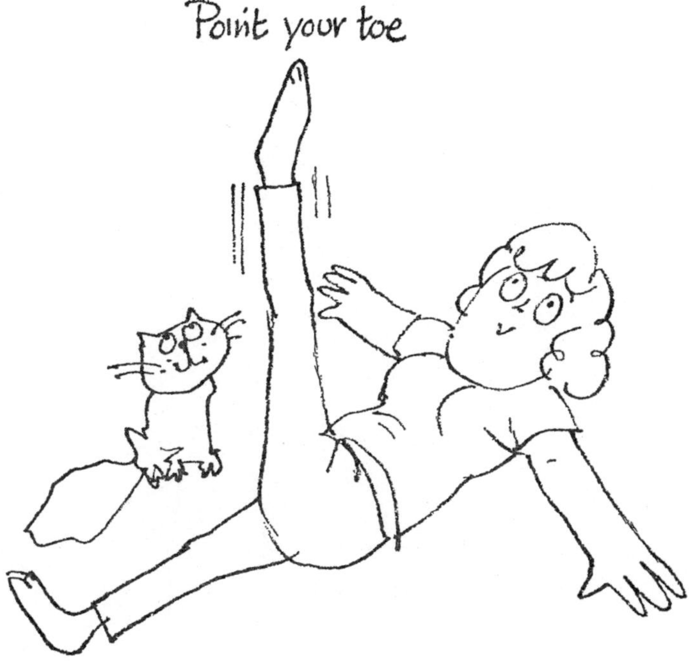

## **44** Stomach and thighs **2**

Get down on to the floor.

Kneel on one knee, kneel on two knees,
lower your body and place your right
hand on the floor to your right side, sit
on your right side, and bring your legs
round so that they are flat on the floor
straight out in front of you. Keep your
back straight. Keeping your foot flat
on the floor as you do so, bend your
right knee towards your chest. Now
hold your knee and your shin with both
hands and try to pull your leg in towards
you.

Put your right knee down and repeat
with your left leg.

Stop if you feel any strain in your
stomach or leg muscles. Try this
exercise, if you can, five times each
leg to begin with and gradually increase.

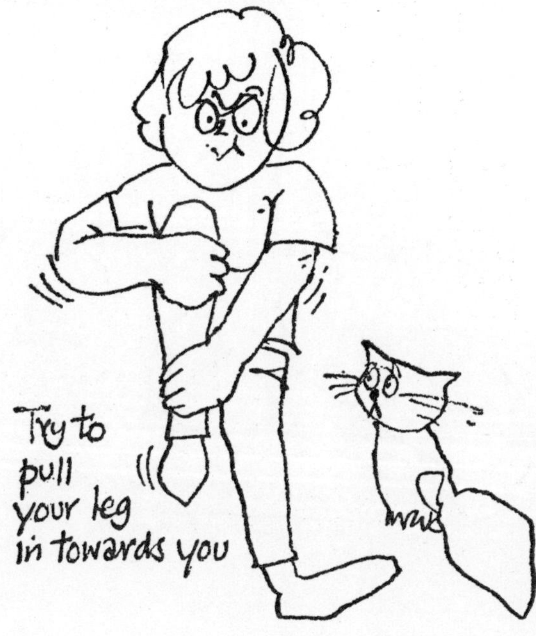

# **45** Back and thigh muscles

Sit on the floor, legs together straight
out in front of you.

Raise your arms above your head,
slowly lower them forward and try to
touch your toes with your fingertips.
Keep your knees straight and if you
point your toes towards the ceiling you
will find this exercise a little easier, as
you haven't got so far to reach!

If you are not used to exercising, you
will probably need some practice before
you can touch your toes.

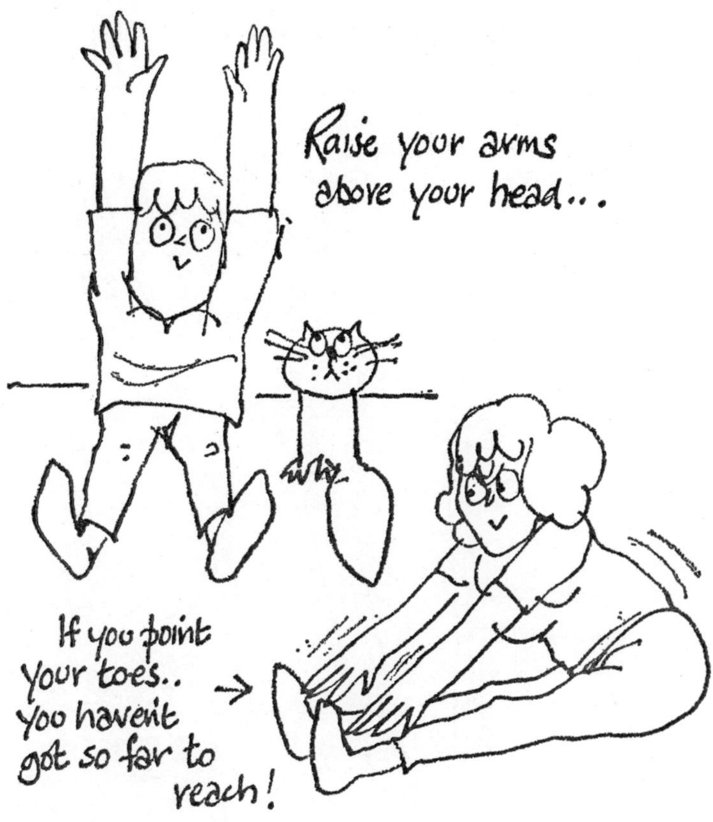

## 46 Thigh muscles 1

For this exercise you will need to use a
chair-back or something solid to hold on
to.

Stand sideways by the chair and hold on
to the back with your right hand.

Swing your right leg straight up in front
of you and swing it straight back.
Repeat this.

Now use your left leg, swing it straight
up in front of you and swing back.

Repeat.

See how high you can kick, but do
keep your leg straight!

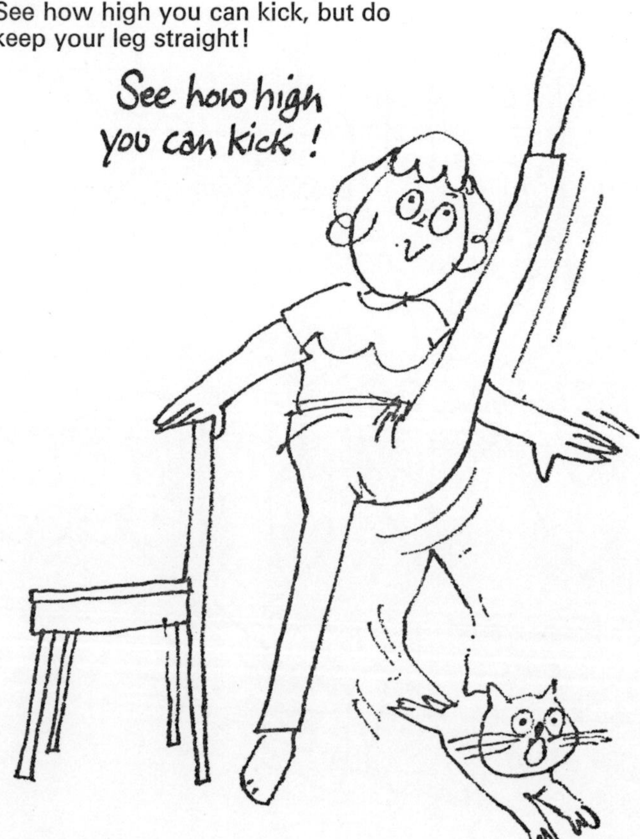

## **47** Thigh muscles 2

Get down on to the floor, then lie flat
on your back with the palms of your
hands face downwards at your side.

Pressing on the palms of your hands,
raise your legs in the air and then
support yourself with the palms of your
hands in the small of your back, so that
your bottom is off the floor.

Your legs should now be straight up in
the air ready to start the pedalling
movement.

Start pedalling slowly, and then build
up speed. Or try making larger wheels
with your legs.

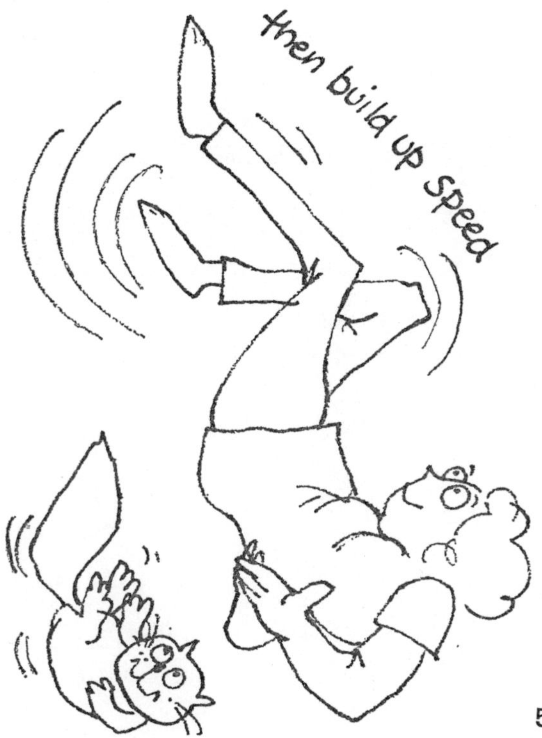

## **48** The thighs **1**

Lie on your right side, legs straight out.
Prop your head comfortably with your
right hand and put your left hand on the
floor in front of you to steady yourself.

Without bending your left leg, raise it
straight up in the air as high as possible.
Lower and repeat six times.

Now turn over on to your left side and
raise your right leg six times.

If you feel any strain, you must of course
stop.

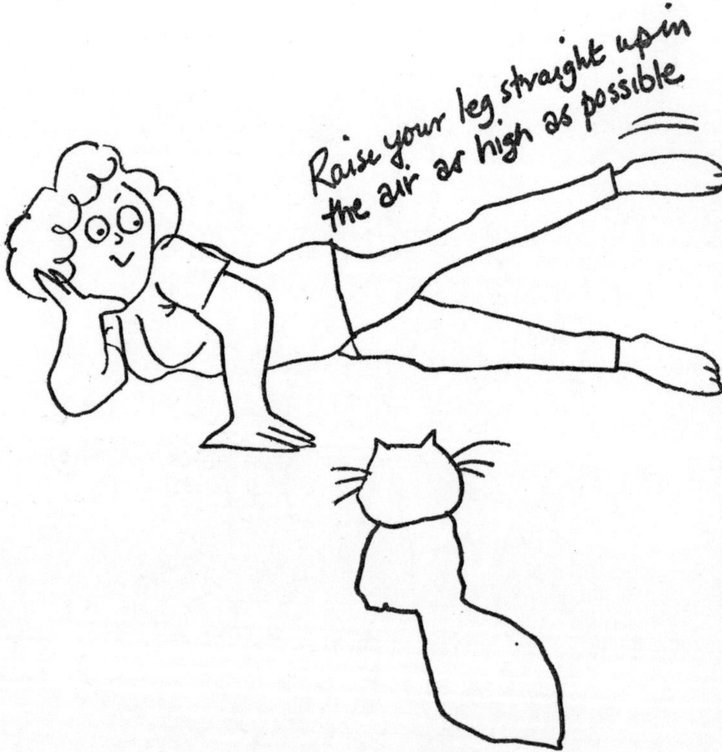

# 49 The thighs 2

Lie flat on your back, hands comfortably at your side, keeping your legs straight.

Raise your right leg straight up in the air, at the same time bringing your arms up, and clap your hands behind your knee. Lower your right leg and repeat with the left. Make sure you keep your legs straight.

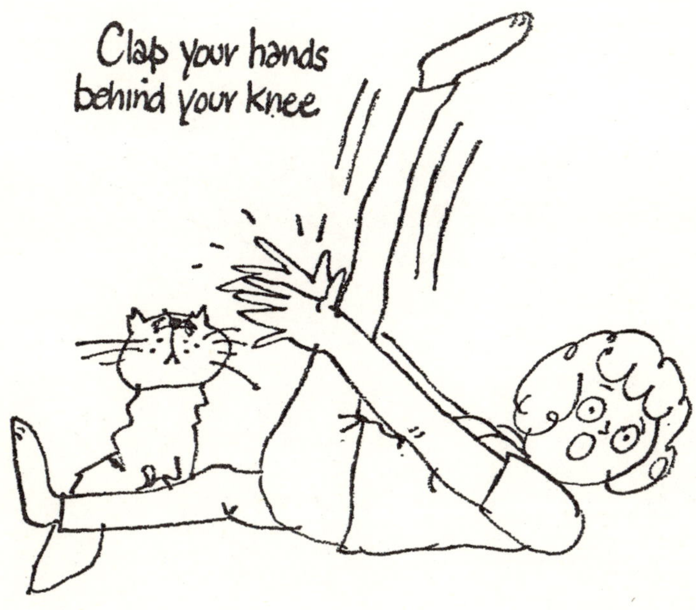

## **50** Thigh lift

For this exercise, you must use the back
of a dining-room chair (or something
similar) to hold on to.

Standing sideways on, hold on to the
back of the chair, keeping your back
straight.

Starting with your right leg, lift and bend
your knee towards your chest. Put down
and repeat with left leg.

This is a very simple exercise and in
order to achieve the best results, you
must remember to keep your back
straight and your stomach in.

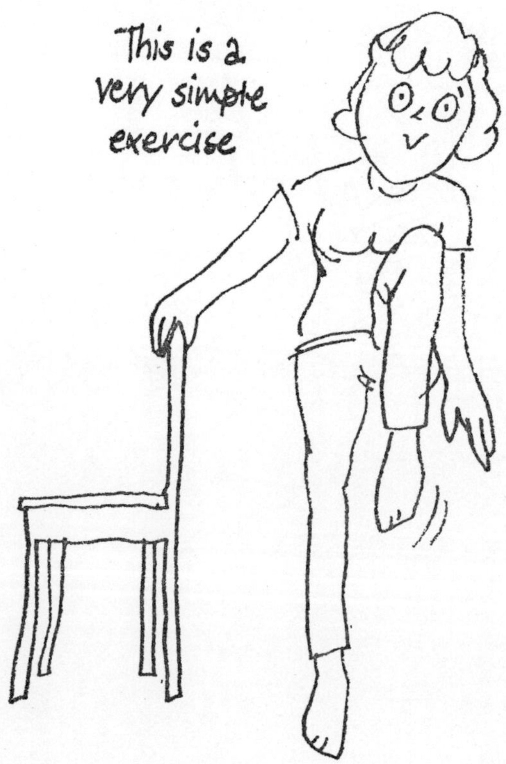

# 51 Thigh muscles

Sit on the floor, legs straight out in front. Place your hands firmly on the floor to the side of you.

Keeping your right leg straight, lift it and swing it as far over to the left as you can. Put it down, rest, then lift it back and put it down straight. Repeat with left leg.

This is a good exercise for thigh muscles if you give a good swing of the leg and get it right over.

Remember to exercise with care, if you are using muscles not normally used.

Take it easy at first. Start with three lifts on each leg and, of course, stop as soon as you feel any strain.

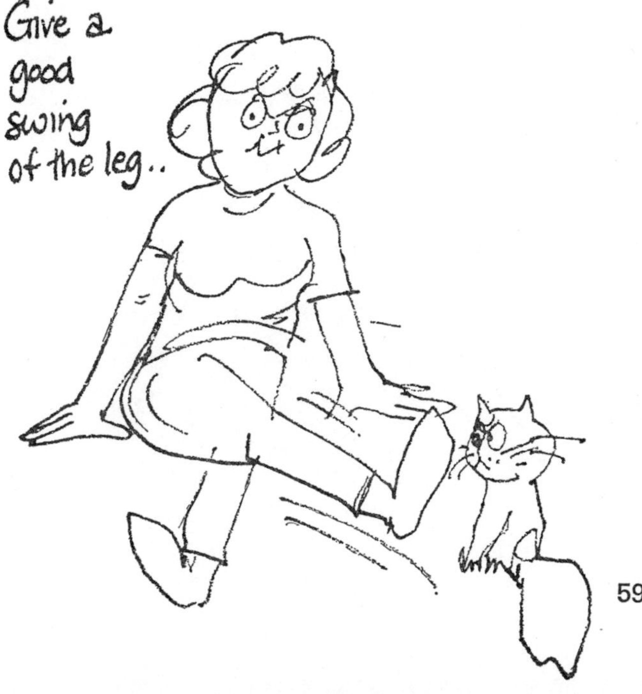

# **52** Hips and thighs

Sit on the floor, legs straight in front.
Raise your knees towards your chin,
keeping feet flat on the floor. Place your
hands firmly on the floor, slightly to
the back of you. Raise your right leg
straight up – *do not bend* – put it down
and raise left leg.

If you do this exercise properly, you
should feel a pull on the muscles at the
back of your thigh.

You may like to start doing this exercise
half a dozen times a day (three lifts on
each leg) and very gradually increase,
but the moment you feel any strain you
must stop.

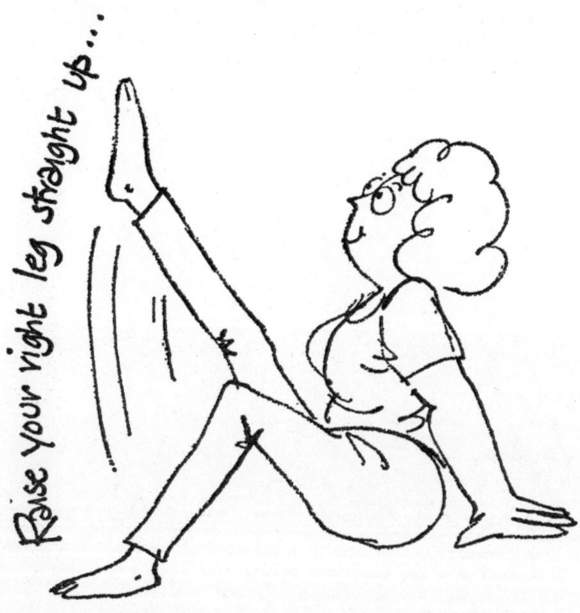

## 53 Bottom, upper arms and shoulders

Lie flat on the floor. Your head, shoulders, back, legs and heels should be touching the floor. Put your arms close to your sides, resting your hands flat on the floor with palms face down.

Push on the palms of your hands and raise your bottom from the floor, still keeping your head, shoulders and heels firmly on the floor.

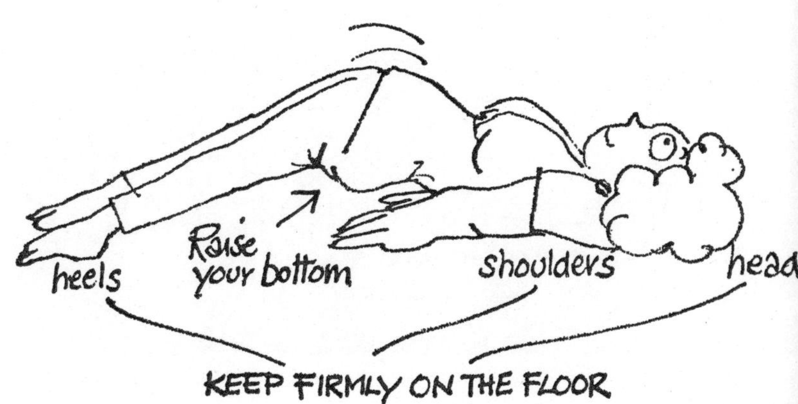

## **54** Bottom, stomach and back

Sit on the floor. Put your legs out in
front, knees straight, and arms straight
out in front.

Use alternately the right arm then the
left, and pull yourself forward, gripping
on an imaginary rope as if you were a
sailor.

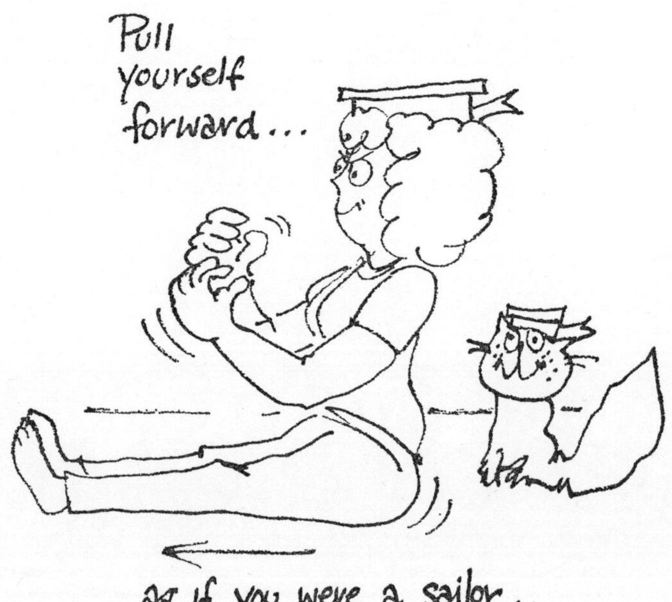

# 55 Hips, legs and ankles

You will need a dining-room chair with no arms and a straight back for this exercise.

Stand facing the chair, feet together.

Bend slightly and take hold of the sides of the chair seat, but keep your legs straight at this stage.

Bend both knees together and go down until you are sitting on your heels. Now straighten up.

Repeat five times to begin with but stop if you feel any strain.

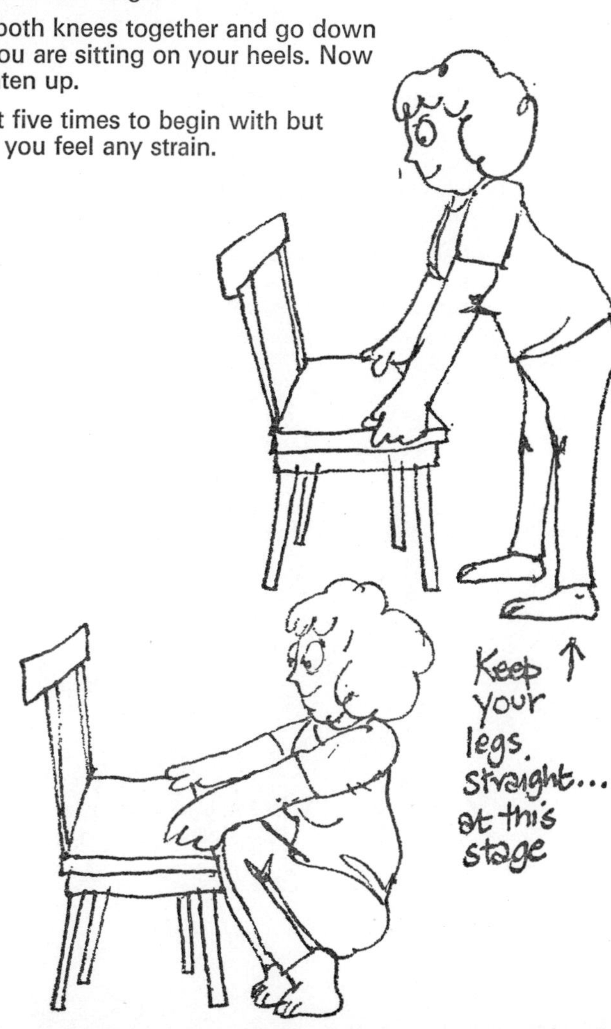

# 56 Leg muscles

Begin your exercise by standing well.

Extend your right foot about three feet
in front of you and turn your right foot
slightly out. Your left leg should be
straight out at the back of you with your
left foot slightly turned out. Place both
of your hands, one on top of the other,
palms face downwards, just above and
on your right knee.

Now press with your hands and let
your right knee bend, still keeping your
left leg straight out behind you.

See how far you can bend your right
knee so that your body becomes lower
to the floor.

It is important with this exercise to keep
your head up and your back straight.
Try this exercise three times on each
leg to begin with, but stop if you feel
any strain.

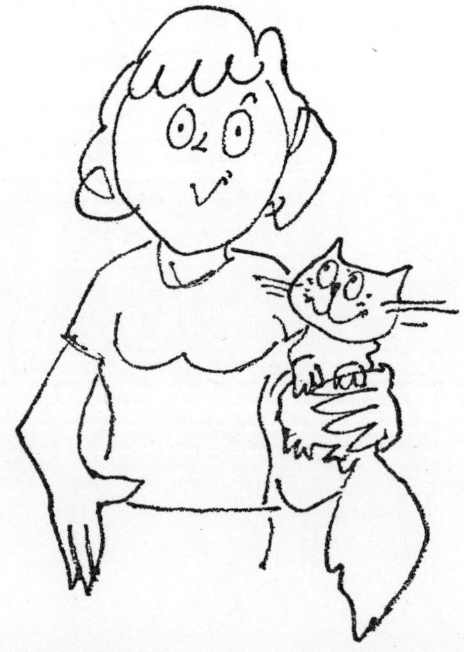